BEAUTY

To James,

Forever grateful for your unconditional support from the beginning.

Hope you enjoy it!

Much love,

Carlota R-B

01. 05. 20

BEAUTY

AS IT IS

CARLOTA RODRIGUEZ-BENITO

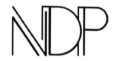

NEW DEGREE PRESS

COPYRIGHT © 2019 CARLOTA RODRIGUEZ-BENITO

BEAUTY

As It Is

ISBN

978-1-64137-313-5   *Paperback*

978-1-64137-606-8   *Ebook*

To Lyle,

for always making sense of my nonsense.

CONTENTS

INTERVIEWEES   13

PROLOGUE   27

HOW TO USE THIS BOOK   31

INTRODUCTION   35

PART I   **HOW WE PERCEIVE**   **39**

CHAPTER 1   WE ALL WANT TO BE BEAUTIFUL   41

                Three Functions of Beauty   41

                A Little History   47

                Where Is Beauty Found?   55

                No Better Cosmetic   57

                Reassess What Beauty Means to You   62

CHAPTER 2   YOUR PERCEPTION OF BEAUTY   65

                Beauty Does Not Equal Sex Appeal   66

                Is Beauty in The Eye of
                the Beholder? Not Exactly   68

Testimonials from Those
Who Work in the Industry   72
What Do They Actually Think?   73
How Different Are These Perceptions Really?   86
Perception of Beauty from
the Regional Perspective   87
Do Some Cultures Inherently Feel More
Beautiful Than Others?   97

PART II   **WHAT WE PRACTICE**   **103**
CHAPTER 3   SUBCONSCIOUSLY SUBSCRIBING TO
             TRENDS, BEHAVIORS AND EXPECTATIONS   105
             What This Industry Is Made Of   107
             Generations: Can We Keep Up with Them All?   114
             Conscious of Trends We Keep Up With   121
             We Have the Power to Choose—
             Take Advantage of It   133

CHAPTER 4   INCLUDING ALL IN THE CONVERSATION   135
             It's a Journey   136
             The Beauty Industry Is onto Something 138
             VOGUE Makes Revolutionary Breakthrough   139
             A Voice of Hope. A Voice of
             Power. A Voice of Beauty.   143
             Public Reaction   147
             The 360° View of Beauty   149
             Diversity and Inclusion   150
             Bridging the Gap   156
             "Don't Hate Me Because I'm Beautiful" 157
             Boys, Boys, Boys   158
             Getting Men's Attention   161

Why So Anti-Aging?   164

Top Inclusive Brands in All Regions   168

CHAPTER 5   CONNECTING WITH YOURSELF AND THE RIGHT INGREDIENTS   173

Feeling Beautiful Is Directly Related to Your Health   173

Holistic Approach   176

Ayurveda: An Old Science becoming the "New Science"   181

Ayurvedic Influence on Today's Wellness Craze   186

Healthy Complexion of the Skin   190

Practicing Safe Beauty   190

Caution: Greenwashing   194

Be Conscious of What You Are Putting on Your Skin   200

Collagen—The Hot Topic   207

Huge "No-Nos"   209

About FDA Legislation   211

Do Some Digging   215

CHAPTER 6   INFLUENCED TO BE A "HACKABLE HUMAN"   219

Two Sides to Every Coin   219

Opening Our Minds   221

Digital Dictatorship   225

Sweet, Sweet, Photoshop   227

They Say, We Do   228

Too Much Trust   232

The Comfort Syndrome   235

Emotionally Attached to Digital Content   240

We Think Influencers Are Our Best Friends   245

PART III   **HOW WE SUCCEED**   **253**

CHAPTER 7   HONOR YOURSELF   255

Digital Life: Down a Rabbit Hole   256

Work Life: As Women in the Workforce   264

Work Life: A Hindu Woman in STEM   267

Work Life: Black Woman Radiating

Beauty on Wall Street   269

Work Life: Own Your Hair   272

Personal Life: Self-Care Is

"In," Take Advantage of It!   276

My Personal Take   278

CHAPTER 8   POWER OF UNIQUE BEAUTY   281

Just Be Yourself   283

OWN IT   286

Express Yourself, Use That Inner Creativity   287

Have Fun with It   291

Can You Maintain Your Unique Beauty with

Cosmetic Treatments or Procedures?   292

No Need for a Mirror   294

More Accessible Than Ever   297

Three Main Consumers   301

The Shift from Reparative to Preventative   304

Hooked on "The Look"   307

Signature Feature   309

CHAPTER 9   THREE BEAUTIES MAKING A DIFFERENCE

IN A SECTOR THEY DIDN'T EXPECT   313

Jeanette Wagner   314

Anastasia Soare   327

Dr. Barbara Sturm   333

PART IV   **A TANGIBLE GIFT FROM THEM TO YOU**   **345**

CHAPTER 10   BECOMING A SMARTER BEAUTY CONSUMER 347

Skin Comes First   348

The Irony!   354

Ingredients That Are Worth the Investment   355

Eat Quality Ingredients as Well   358

Twelve-Step Routine Not Needed!   361

Don't Be a Victim of Greenwashing!   365

Toxic "ness" and Clean "ness"   366

Quality = $$$?   369

Ayurvedic Beauty Routines   373

Clear through the Noise   375

We Care about Sustainability and Efficiency   377

CHAPTER 11   SUCCEED IN YOUR BEAUTY BUSINESS   381

A Life Dedicated to Your Passion   382

Blurred Lines: Work and Personal Life   384

But Really, Do Your Homework   386

Consumer-Centric Beauty   387

Beauty Branding   388

Communicating Your Story to
Different Markets   396

Is Too Saturated a Bad Thing?   404

What Constitutes Success?   406

EPILOGUE   409

WORKS REFERENCED   413

ACKNOWLEDGMENTS   421

INTERVIEWEES

—

Anastasia Soare is the founder, CEO, and driving force behind Anastasia Beverly Hills—one of the fastest-growing brands in the beauty industry. In 1990, she introduced a new brow shaping technique to clients—later patented as the Golden Ratio Eyebrow Shaping Method—that has gone on to become a modern beauty essential. Anastasia is a beauty pioneer and powerhouse.

Anne Booth Dayton is the Director of Institutional Advancement at El Museo del Barrio and previously was the Chief Operating Officer at Collectrium, a Christie's Company.

Arden Martin is a teacher of Vedic Meditation and co-founder of The Spring Meditation Studio in New York City. She cares deeply about bringing more transparency to the US personal care industry and works with Beautycounter to educate people about what "clean beauty" really means.

Ariane Hunter is the CEO and founder of Project She Went For Her Dreams—a personal branding and marketing firm in New York City, serving clients globally. She works with enlightened women and businesses to develop creative brands and build artistic marketing strategies to stand out in a meaningful, authentic way.

Dr. Ava Shamban is the owner and director of two branded practices—AVA MD, her full-service Dermatology clinics in Santa Monica, Beverly Hills, and new concept SKINFIVE in West LA/Century City and Pacific Palisades. She is a renowned board-certified dermatologist, true skin visionary, clinician, author, anti-aging expert, prejuvenation proponent, and now co-host on The GIST Show.

Dr. Barbara Sturm is the founder and CEO of Dr. Barbara Sturm Molecular Cosmetics. She is a German aesthetics doctor, widely renowned for her anti-inflammatory philosophy and her non-surgical anti-aging skin treatments. Dr. Sturm translated science from her clinical research and orthopedic practice into the field of aesthetics and has been a success ever since.

Bisila Bokoko is the founder and CEO of BBES, a business development agency in New York that represents and promotes international market brands. She has inspired thousands of people and organizations around the world through conferences in which she has motivated others to pursue dreams, think big, and talk about empowerment, entrepreneurship, geopolitics, and personal branding.

Chinwe Esimai is the Managing Director and Chief Anti-Bribery Officer at Citigroup, Inc. She is also an award-winning lawyer, author, and speaker who is passionate about inspiring generations of immigrant women leaders.

Clémence von Mueffling is the Founder and Editor of Beauty and Well-Being (BWB), which brings a fresh aesthetic to the beauty and well-being media. She is also the author of *Ageless Beauty the French Way*, a luxurious, entertaining, unparalleled guide to every French beauty secret for all women.

Ewelina Aiossa is the Assistant Vice President of Marketing at SkinCeuticals, L'Oreal. She serves on UBM—Dermatology Times Industry Council and SkinCeuticals (SC) Leadership Team panel. She has a strong knowledge of the aesthetic business, professional channel, products, and ingredients.

Fleur Phelipeau is the CEO and Founder of D-LAB Nutricosmetics, Birdie Nutrition, and Claude Aphrodisiacs. She has surrounded herself with doctors from Vichy Célestins ever since she was a little girl, which played a huge role in her innate affinity for hyper-nutrition beauty from within. Nutricosmetics are Fleur's passion; she has been working with them for over fifteen years.

Franck Moison is the former Chief Operating Officer and Vice Chairman of Colgate-Palmolive. He is an experienced Non-Executive Director with a demonstrated history of working in the consumer goods industry.

Georg von Griesheim is CEO of Health & Beauty, where they offer events for the manufacturing of cosmetic products, international distribution, and platforms to the professional user in a joint venture with Germany's leading people's magazine to the final consumer.

Hannah Cecille is currently a Creative Producer for the largest account on the platform (@Instagram). She is an empathetic storyteller and host who believes it is her purpose to share the stories of underrepresented communities in the world.

Jacinda Heintz is an Influencer Marketing Coordinator at Kendo Brands, Inc. She leverages her social media and marketing expertise to create socially driven partnerships that are mutually beneficial for both the brand and the influencer.

Jeanette Wagner is the Vice Chairman Emerita of The Estée Lauder Companies Inc. Mrs. Wagner joined the Estée Lauder

Companies as the Vice President, Director of Marketing of the Estée Lauder brand in the International Division. In that role, she revolutionized the process of bringing products to market and exploded the growth of the Lauder brand internationally. She is also Chairman CEO of Nulli Secundus Associates, a pro bono consulting company.

Jeanne Chavez is the President and co-founder of the beauty brands, Smith & Cult, and the co-founder of Hard Candy. She has had a decades-long career in beauty, starting off at Orlane Institute to luxury brand La Prairie before ending up at her current position.

Jenny Villasana is a top certified Life Coach, Author of Children's books, and Radio Talk Show Host at *El Carrousel de tus Sueños* / Cadena Azul 1550 am.

Jordana Shiau is a Manager of Social and Digital Strategy at Laura Mercier. She has been in the corporate side of the beauty industry for the last five years working from startups to the largest beauty brands in the world.

Dr. John Martin is a Harvard-educated Medical Doctor who specializes in Facial Cosmetic Surgery as well as other non-surgical treatment for vascular and pigment problems as well as skin rejuvenation. Dr. Martin has been featured in *The Doctors, The Dr. Oz Show, Dr. Phil,* and *Anderson Cooper 360°*.

Dr. Jouhayna Alouie is a well-known esthetician in Beirut, Paris, and Riyadh, who has been working in the field since the mid-seventies. She specializes in corrective work, permanent makeup, and enhancement facial treatments. In the past, she has worked closely with Miss France and many Arab celebrities.

Karla Martinez de Salas is the Editor-in-Chief for *Vogue Mexico and Latin America*. She was recently included in the Business of Fashion (BoF) US list of the five hundred international fashion leaders, and since then, Karla has been in charge of the magazine's management. *Vogue Mexico and Latin America* was also awarded with best editorial content by Mexico's Fashion Digital Awards.

Kennedy Daniel works part time at Glossier LA on Melrose Place as an Offline Editor while she finishes her BA at the University of Southern California. Kennedy is proud to say she was a member of the original team of Offline Editors who helped open the store in the Spring of 2018.

Klara Chrzuszcz is a Medical Skin care Aesthetician, Clinical Skin care Expert, and the owner of Klara Beauty Lab. Klara is an educator in Europe for neurotoxin application as well as dermal fillers for the face and body, and she travels to teach on a yearly basis. Her approach involves delving into clients' lifestyles, diets, stress levels, etc. which, allows her to create a one-of-a-kind experience.

Dr. Lauren Hazzouri is a licensed psychologist, international public speaker, founder of Hazzouri Psychology, Scranton, and founder of NOT THERAPY—a program she created to address the unique mental health concerns of girls and women. She has been named one of the "Top 5 Women in the World Inspiring Girls" by German *Glamour,* and her trailblazing work has appeared in publications including *Teen Vogue, Forbes,* and British *Vogue.*

Maria Calderon is the CEO and founder of Kosmetai, founder of Institut Nahia, and founder of Juveskin, S.L. company, where she serves as Director General and is the Technical Director of PRODUCTOS BIORGANICOS, S.L. Maria is a chemical cosmetic pharmaceutical specialist and licensed expert in the evaluation of the security and information files of cosmetic products.

Maria Eugenia Leon is the protagonist of "Blogger en Exclusiva," the Director and founder of the famous Spanish beauty blog, *Belleza en Vena,* and co-founder of *El Club de Las 11.* She writes honestly and transparently about cosmetics, perfumes, personal care, decoration, and much more.

Marie Englesson is now working as a retail and supply chain consultant in the East African region. Prior, she started up her own beauty retail and distribution business in Tanzania, called Atsoko. Starting from scratch, she developed a retail platform with seven stores and introduced twelve global beauty brands in the market. In early 2018, when she sold her business, Atsoko was ranked among the top one hundred medium-sized companies in Tanzania.

Meghna Chakraborty is now a graduate student at the University of Southern California. Previously, she was a content strategy intern at Live Tinted, a multicultural beauty brand. Driven by her passion for innovative experiences and diverse storytelling, she is determined to help elevate unheard voices and underrepresented faces in media and pop culture.

Mi Anne Chan is an Associate Producer and Staff Writer at Refinery29, a video director at Condé Nast entertainment, and a beauty influencer/vlogger. She has been writing, editing, filming, and making tutorials on all things beauty related since the start of her career.

Nayera Senane is a Diamond Allergan Injector, Botox and dermal filler expert. She currently holds a wide client base including celebrities and models. Although based in Los Angeles, she travels regularly to the East Coast to see clients.

Nihar Neelakanti is an investor at Kauffman Fellows Fund, produces The Arena Podcast, and writes the Journal Newsletter by Kauffman Fellows. Previously, he was an analyst at Correlation Ventures, which has invested in notable consumer companies such as Casper, Cotopaxi, and Imperfect Produce. He also cofounded Vendima Bags, a direct-to-consumer luxury bag startup.

Olga Lorencin is the owner of Olga Lorencin Skin Care Clinic and CEO and founder for Olga Lorencin Skin Care. She is a top-tier esthetician and skin care guru and has spent more than twenty years in the treatment room studying ingredients. Olga is affectionately referred to as "The Acid Queen."

Olivier Lechère is the General Director for Chanel Spain & Portugal in charge of the three divisions: Fashion, Fragrance & Beauty and Watches & Fine Jewelry in Madrid. He has dedicated these last twenty years to driving and growing the business by setting up two fashion flagship stores, boosting the fragrances and beauty division to number one in the Spanish market.

Paty De San Román is the co-founder of Brand Dreamers and has been a communications and PR consultant specialized in beauty, fashion, health and lifestyle for fifteen years. She has worked on campaigns La Roche-Posay, Maria Duol, Grupo Marchon, and many others. Paty is a dreamer herself and loves communicating ideas to the greater public.

Peter Thomas Roth is the CEO, founder, and formulator of Peter Thomas Roth Clinical Skin Care, is an influential segment leader in the beauty industry and continues to corner the clinical market as a groundbreaking, results-focused innovator. Today, Peter's comprehensive range of products are sold worldwide in over eighty countries, with Peter leading all research and development efforts at his state-of-the-art lab and manufacturing facility.

Priyanka Chopra Jonas is an Indian actress, model, singer, and film producer who began her fame when she won the Miss World 2000 pageant.

Roya Pourshalchi is a dedicated yoga teacher, Ayurveda consultant at Kilona Shop, and Marma bodywork therapist. Roya currently sees clients privately and hosts group classes and workshops in New York City. She is Yoga Alliance RYT-200 certified, trained in 100 HR Ayurveda Foundations and 100 HR Marma Therapy.

Dr. Sami Helou is one of the most renowned specialized plastic surgeons in Beirut, Lebanon.

Shadoh Punnapuzha is the Founder of Taïla Skincare. She is proving that when you combine the power of Ayurveda and science, you get divine results. After years of working at a PE firm in NYC and going through a burnout, Shadoh found her path to a healthy life and a healthy skin through Ayurveda.

Stephanie Peterson is a model and the founder of Smoothie Beauty, a clean and organic skin care line that is truly fresh without any toxic chemicals, additives, or preservatives. She is also the creator of The Global Beauty blog. She has modeled in more than fifteen countries, with the likes of Clinique, Mary Kay and Pandora, among others.

Susana Martinez Vidal is a journalist and author, founder of *Ragazza* magazine, which catapulted her to becoming the youngest director of any edition of *Elle* in the world. After seeing the first exhibit of Frida Kahlo's clothing at the Casa Azul in 2012, she was inspired to write her first book, *Frida Kahlo: Fashion as the Art of Being*, recommended by *The New York Times* and *Vanity Fair UK*—most important magazines in more than twenty countries.

Teresa De La Cierva is an excellent journalist and communicator, working for ABC writing about beauty for almost her entire career. She started writing on paper and then created one of the first five blogs in the newspaper, called "La Polvera," which was about beauty. She is frequently featured speaking about beauty on Federico Jiménez Losantos' radio show on esRadio's Morning.

Tyle Mahoney is an expert colorist with more than fifteen years of experience at MèCHE salon. Clients depend on him not only for his skill when it comes to creating the perfect color, but also for his ability to make his creations last. Considering lifestyle as well as the elements, Tyle tailors his methods to ensure fade-resistant color and shine. He works hand in hand with Tracey Cunningham.

Valentina Collado Rojas is the Fashion Editor and Stylist of *Vogue Mexico & Latin America*. She was previously an Assistant for Special Events Department at Vogue Condé Nast Americas. She is experienced in Editorial and Fashion Styling, Event Planning, Online/New Media, PR, and Sales industries.

Yalda Alaoui is the Founder of Eat Burn Sleep. Yalda was diagnosed in 2007 with two auto-immune diseases—Ulcerative Colitis and Auto-Immune Haemolytic Anaemia—that made her begin to extensively research nutrition and health. A ten-year period of research and recovery led her to share her knowledge and make a full career change in order to help more people.

Yalitza Aparicio is a Mexican actress who made her film debut as Cleo in Alfonso Cuarón's 2018 drama, *Roma*, which earned her a nomination for an Academy Award for Best Actress. *Time* magazine named her one of the one hundred most influential people in the world in 2019.

Yolanda Sactristán is the General Director of TheBeautyNewsroom.com and the former Editor-in-Chief of renowned publications: *Vogue* (2001-2017) and *Harper's Bazaar* (2017-2019). Yolanda is a skilled journalist with a passion for fashion, beauty, and luxury. She is always determined to produce compelling stories.

PROFESSIONALS WHO REQUESTED TO REMAIN ANONYMOUS:

A Generation Z beauty connoisseur and university student and influencer from Hong Kong

A professional in the cosmetic fillers sphere who works for a leading global pharmaceutical company

A professional in the medical aesthetic industry

A well-known nutritionist and holistic beauty practitioner in Los Angeles

A young woman who shares about her experience with toxic beauty forums

The Chief Marketing Officer at a leading multinational beauty company

The Global Executive Director of Digital Education at a leading brand of multinational beauty company

The Head of EMEA beauty business of a leading multinational corporation

The Head of LATAM at a leading multinational beauty company

The Head of Marketing LATAM at a multinational beauty company

The Head of the Greater China beauty business at a leading multinational corporation

The Marketing Director of the Americas beauty division at a luxury goods company

The Vice President of Global Marketing at a world leading beauty company

The Vice President of Greater China beauty business at a leading multinational corporation

PROLOGUE

———

When I told my mother I was going to write this book, she showed me a hysterical home video from when I was about three or four years old. I was wearing chic white sunglasses and watching *Sleeping Beauty* on the arm of my living room couch, all while painting my toenails with an eyeshadow palette and brush. I was immersed in the movie, paying little to no attention to the outcome of the eyeshadow pedicure I was giving myself. While I might not have known the right place to put the eyeshadow, I did uncover an innate love for beauty from a young age.

My mother was never a beauty buff, yet anyone who meets her can easily mistake her for a guru. She never painted her nails while I was growing up, nor did she expose me to any of the products and beauty tendencies I was constantly drawn to during my teenage years; it came from elsewhere. Aside from the occasional lip liner, blush, and under-eye cover up, she always embraced a very natural look, placing far more emphasis on caring for her inner beauty and cultivating her love for healthy Mediterranean recipes.

On the other hand, my "abuelitas"[1] adored fashion and all things glamorous. For those of you who do not know much about Bilbao, Spain, where my whole family is from, they were what you would call "Señoras de Las Arenas" aka, the notoriously most put together, in style, and elegant women in all of Bilbao.

The influences of these three amazing women, my mother and two grandmothers, paired with my prima ballerina background, became the springboard for my fascination in beauty and its origin.

Perhaps just as impactful as the aforementioned ladies is my father's profession's constant requirement for relocation. Thanks to the constant moves, both by intention and by necessity, I am fluent in Spanish, Russian, French, and English. Yet, I found none of these to be sufficient in communicating the message of beauty. With nonverbal communication beauty can be fully captivated: the way we carry

---

1   What I called my grandmothers in Spanish.

ourselves, our confidence, our openness, our knowledge, our self-esteem. You get the point.

The journey in composing this book has not only granted me a great level of fulfillment, but also left me room for self-reflection. Through conversations with beauty professionals, I find myself constantly revisiting my own definition of beauty and, at times, coming to peace with my own personal insecurities. It has been, and I speculate it is a rite of passage, a constant battle with imposter syndrome to think I am now a published author. It is not the "Wows" or pride that spur me on, but rather, the chance to partake in open dialogue with all of you.

HOW TO USE THIS BOOK

———

Each chapter can be read as a standalone. Hence a completed visit is not needed to extract the book's core message.

WHAT IS ITS PURPOSE?

My hope is that, in reading *Beauty as It Is*, you will discover inspiring accounts from sixty plus elite professionals in the skin care and cosmetics industries from around the world. This book is a tool to position the beauty business in your mind as a means of empowerment and not as a means to hide your true self. Lastly, I hope for people in the beauty business to learn from accounts of high-end professionals, in order to achieve success in today's increasingly saturated beauty world.

This book is meant to bring an idea to light that for some might be eye-opening, and to others, blatantly obvious. It is about sharing a perception of beauty that can be more holistic, honest, transparent, and unique to each individual's lifestyle.

Each chapter comes back to highlight the importance of self-exploration and finding what gives you the confidence to *feel* beautiful and not only "look" beautiful—because as you will learn by reading, no one really knows what "looking beautiful" means.

Ultimately, I want you to feel that you are seated right next to me, interviewing the professionals. I want you to feel that they are talking to YOU. With all their fascinating stories, I hope you gain a panoramic view of what the industry looks like today, gaining an awareness of beauty trends, ingredients, and innovations.

THE BOOK IS AT THE INTERSECTION OF FOUR THEMES:

- Global shifts in the perception of beauty
- New trends in consumer behavior
- Best practices for new and existing beauty brands and businesses
- Best practices and things to know for the curious beauty consumer

YOU WILL LOVE THIS BOOK IF YOU ARE INTERESTED IN:

- Re-assessing your own perception of beauty
- Getting an inside view into the conversations and trends that are occurring within the beauty industry
- Learning from *crème de la crème* beauty professionals
- Becoming a more conscious beauty consumer
- Becoming a more informed beauty business leader

YOU WILL ENJOY THIS BOOK IF YOU ARE A BEAUTY:

- Consumer
- Innovator
- Executive
- Marketer
- Editor
- Blogger
- Influencer

WHAT TO KEEP IN MIND?

As you read, you may notice professionals' names used throughout the book with no explanation of where they work or additional context. This is an intentional stylistic approach to avoid having to interrupt content by repeating who each person is, as they may appear multiple times in the book in different chapters. Instead, I have footnoted both the company and position of all the individuals I have interviewed, heard, or read about throughout other sources.

Some of the professionals, due to legal reasons with their companies, have chosen to remain anonymous.

Additionally, throughout the book I mention brands and companies. I would like to clarify that I am in no way affiliated or connected with those brands and do not receive monetary gain by mentioning them. Information on the brands will be placed in footnotes as well to prevent distraction from content.

INTRODUCTION

While I am originally from Spain, I grew up living in the US, Switzerland, Mexico, Spain, France, and Russia. Being raised in different cultures, belief systems, and world views while attending international schools, the question of how different societies around the world perceive, feel, and consume beauty intrigued me.

It interested me to know what it was about beauty that gave so much power to certain people.

Was it the way they walked, talked, or carried themselves?

What allowed these people to radiate so much beauty no matter what they looked like?

When I lived in Switzerland, I specifically remember a woman who had a presence that exuded *je ne sais quoi,* making her beauty unparalleled. Although her genetic makeup was nothing out of the ordinary, she was enthralling. The minute she walked into one of the dinner parties my parents would host, all eyes were on her. I remember wondering, *Why? Others had the potential to be just as radiant as her, but they weren't.* Now, I understand what this woman had was complete control of her inner beauty and how to project it outward. This woman had mastered the art of *feeling* beautiful.

For me, my confidence in my own beauty came from my extensive exposure to the stage. I learned I had to *feel* beautiful in order to be perceived as beautiful by the audience. My ballet teachers were the ones who taught me the importance of *feeling* beautiful, as all ballerinas are trained to strive for this feeling.

The life of a ballerina is not in any sense luxurious or filled with beauty, but it certainly taught me to radiate as much of my inner beauty as possible with every single movement in order to captivate the attention of the audience.

Although there are endless nuances to the perception of beauty in each region of the world, something undoubtedly remains the same—your physical self is only the vehicle through which you transmit your inner beauty. Both forms of beauty, physical and inner, are important in their respective ways. But, without something valuable on the inside to transmit outward, our external vessel is useless.

Even the most talented ballerina cannot get lead roles in a ballet unless the crowd can feel the energy and emotion she transmits.

Does this mean, the heck with skin-deep beauty, and people who care about physical beauty are vain?

Absolutely not.

If external beauty is the vehicle to export our inner beauty, we should take care of it too. This is where color cosmetics, cosmetic treatments, and skin care come in.

It is crucial to remember the function of beauty products is to highlight and celebrate your inner beauty, not to hide it.

After all, beauty is a choice. The moment you choose to *feel* beautiful, you are beautiful.

PART I

HOW WE PERCEIVE

CHAPTER 1

WE ALL WANT TO
BE BEAUTIFUL

———

What does it mean to be beautiful?

Is it to be symmetrical, perfect, attractive…? What is it?

THREE FUNCTIONS OF BEAUTY

Dr. Ava Shamban[2] and I were at the Palisades Sunday
Farmers Market in Los Angeles purchasing some fresh

———

2   Dr. Ava Shamban is the owner and director of two branded practices—
AVA MD, her full-service Dermatology clinics in Santa Monica,
Beverly Hills and new concept SKINFIVE in West LA/Century City
and Pacific Palisades. She is a renowned board-certified dermatologist,
true skin visionary, clinician, author, anti-aging expert, prejuvenation
proponent, and now co-host on The GIST Show.

produce before heading to her home to cook up a nice nutritious brunch and talk about the beauty industry. I have to say, normally I always come prepared for sun activities, but here we were. Dr. Shamban was covered head to toe with her nice summer sun-proof wear, hat, and sunscreen while her cousin was just as prepared, and there I was in a skirt, short-sleeve shirt, and no hat protection... I must not have made the best skin-conscious impression on the doctor. I *was* wearing my sunscreen, however. That is an absolute must!

"You've got to find the clear sound," said a sixty-year-old man to Dr. Shamban and me while we tapped all the watermelons in the basket in search of the one with the "clear sound." They say the juicier watermelons sound a certain way.

We indeed found the "clear sound" and perfect watermelon. It seemed like this man had also found something... me. I would be his next target to ask on a date—scary, I know.

After the watermelon encounter, this man continued to approach me throughout the farmers market. He asked me innocent questions like, where I was from, what I was doing in Los Angeles, what I studied in university, why I decided to major in Russian, French and International Relations.... Long story short, this man was having an intermittent conversation with me at the market as we shopped from tent to tent. To me this felt like one of my friends' parents talking to me, being curious, nothing strange or so I thought.

All of a sudden, he asked me, "Would you like to get coffee or a drink with me tomorrow?" I thought, to myself, *Ummmm, say that again?* I was so confused by his proposition that it took me a second to react.

Well, I clearly was not going to do that. However, this man unintentionally taught me a lesson about beauty in this moment. Who would have known what this sixty-year-old man asked me was going to prompt Dr. Shamban to begin the conversation of beauty at its core—the human condition?

I bring up this anecdote because this was a great example of the biological perception of beauty. For this sixty-year-old man, a young twenty-two-year-old could have captured his attention because of the human natural desire to reproduce.

Youth implies fertility. This reveals why we are so obsessed with looking young. It is a subconscious instinct, of which we are often unaware.

Dr. Shamban and I laughed about this encounter afterward— she saw it all happen—and she warned me to be prepared for similar encounters in the future. As we got in the car to go back to her home she said,

So what you just witnessed was one function of beauty. There are three major functions of beauty in my opinion. They are the following:

1. **Sexual Selection:** Humans as a species have a natural instinct to have someone to partner with and perpetuate their genes. It's called sexual selection and was identified by Darwin.

   This phenomenon is present across all animal kingdoms, not only in human beings. What is interesting about this phenomenon in the animal kingdom is that females are the ones that need to be impressed, yet in humans it's the men. I think we humans have gotten it all wrong (she laughs). In the Middle Ages, the men would dress up more. They would wear makeup and heels to show off their calves' musculature. Funny how things change, right?

2. **Nonverbal Communication:** The second component of beauty is communication. Most communication is nonverbal

communication, which is based mostly on people's expressions on their faces and their gestures.

This is why the "Resting Bitch Face" is such a thing. People can communicate a frown, if they are concentrating or thinking about something, and although they are not intentionally making that face, to the observer it does communicate a message of anger, sadness, or boredom.

"Resting Bliss Face" is also a thing, and it's a good thing. It's when you always look happy. You can have a little smile in the corner of your mouth, and you can smile with your eyes.

3. **Facial Feedback Hypothesis:** The third component is the Facial Feedback Hypothesis (FFH), which is a hypothesis that states that emotions can be caused or enhanced depending on your expression or how you see yourself. If you look at yourself in the mirror and you look good, you will smile and feel better. Some people call this a good hair day or a day that you simply think you look good.

So, why is that so?

Why would we care if we looked good or not?

We are genetically programmed to want to look good because that makes our genes more likely to be reproduced. Which brings us back to sexual selection. If we look good, we will score in sexual selection.

What does this have to do with Dr. Shamban's philosophy of beauty?

Years ago Allergan,[3] the leading pharmaceutical company, asked her to give a talk about beauty in Hollywood. In the talk, she said there was a lot of bad cosmetic work being done in Hollywood and people are tampering with their faces. "People in Hollywood were not paying attention to the features in their faces that are already beautiful. I call this their Signature Feature." Her philosophy of Signature Feature was the biggest takeaway from her talk at Allergan and what people most ask her about to this day.

Dr. Ava Shamban says,

> All the work to I do is centered around having mem-
> orable people and allowing their Signature Feature
> to be seen. All Signature Feature means is that some-
> thing about every face out there in the world is very

---

3   Allergan is a pharmaceutical company that owns Botox
    (botulinum toxin), Linzess (linaclotide), Bystolic (nebivolol),
    Juvederm (injectable filler), Latisse (bimatoprost), and many more.

compelling and memorable. This is why engaging with my patients is my favorite part of my job. I'm often told "I hate this, I hate that, I hate such and such about myself." But the way I like to approach my clients is to start from a positive point of view. I like starting the conversation with pointing out their most beautiful striking feature and telling them how they can clear their palette to make that feature pop.

Dr. Shamban has created something special with her coining of the Signature Feature. Most of the time people don't think this way, and they solely focus on the features they are not happy or comfortable with. It is important to work with our Signature Features to keep our uniqueness and authenticity alive.

A LITTLE HISTORY

Now that we have a gist of what our biological need of beauty looks like, how has this manifested through time?

Cosmetic rituals are some of the earliest human culture practices known to us. Despite all the different regions and societies in the world, we all have been caring about beautifying rituals and techniques since the beginning of time. For years, people have craved *feeling* beautiful, and we continue to do so—maybe even more today with so many options, advancements, and easy access to beauty. We can track a fascination as far as 7,000 years ago with the Ancient Greeks, Romans, and Egyptians.[4]

In 51 BC, Cleopatra pioneered makeup and cosmetics, using natural kohl and other ingredients to create her signature eyes.[5] Hygiene and skin care, with rose water and castor oil for example, were also important beauty factors in Egyptian society back then and are still prominent in the beauty world today.

An expert in the history of beauty and Harvard Business School Professor, Geoffrey Jones, agrees with Dr. Shamban. In an interview for a Harvard Business School article he says, "The human desire to attract reflects basic biological motivations. Every human society from at least the ancient Egyptians onwards has used beauty products and artifacts to enhance attractiveness. However, beauty ideals have always varied enormously over time and between societies."[6]

We have been altering our physical looks to *feel* more beautiful for as far as history can remember. Lip and eye pigmentation

4   "Cleopatra's Eye: The Significance of Kohl in Ancient Egypt." 2018. The Recipes Project. Accessed September 30, 2019. https://recipes.hypotheses.org/12837.

5   Ibid.

6   "The History of Beauty." 2010. HBS Working Knowledge. Accessed September 30, 2019. https://hbswk.hbs.edu/item/the-history-of-beauty.

have been used in Iraq since 2000 BC.[7] Foot binding was done in China on girls between ages five and six, so the foot would be made narrower and shorter—a desirable feature for their standard of beauty at the time. This started in the tenth century and lasted until about 1949.[8] Furthermore, from the Renaissance to the nineteenth century, women from many Western cultures also altered the way they looked by using corsets to make them look more beautiful and to fit the standard of beauty of the time. Women in Burma and Thailand also wore and still to this day wear neck rings to elongate their necks to look more beautiful within their society. All of this highlights that all over the world, beauty has been focused on since the beginning of time. It is a way to remain interesting, feel good about ourselves, and make sure we keep our DNA alive.

This really shows that any inclination to enhance our beauty is nothing new, and nothing for which we should feel ashamed.

The Beginning of "The Standard"

In the nineteenth century a homogenization of beauty ideals surfaced. This was specifically targeted more toward Western, fair-skinned women, as the era of Western imperialism

---

7   Ibid.
8   Anne Booth Dayton is the Director of Institutional Advancement at El Museo del Barrio and previously was the Chief Operating Officer at Collectrium, a Christie's Company

was on the rise. "The industry's contribution was to turn these underlying trends into brands, create aspirations that drove their growing use, and then employ modern marketing methods to globalize them," Geoffrey Jones mentions.[9]

Fast forward to the twentieth century, the industrial revolution caused a huge shift in the cosmetics and beauty industry. Cosmetics started to be made for the masses.[10] Interestingly, the Russian ballet introduced color cosmetics to Paris, and then later on to the United States.[11] Ballerinas began the trend of wearing pronounced makeup, so their faces would be visible to those sitting far from the stage.

As a result, people started using makeup in their daily beauty routines. Many women, however, were not accepted or were regarded as sinners if they wore makeup. Over time, it became more acceptable for women to use cosmetics, although it was still predominantly reserved for performers. Fast forward some years, Hollywood culture was one of the largest influencers and had a huge impact on cosmetics, with key figures changing the way we viewed cosmetics forever.

---

9   Ibid.
10 "History of Makeup | History of Cosmetics | BH Cosmetics LLC." 2019. BH Cosmetics. Accessed September 30, 2019. https://www.bhcosmetics.com/pages/resources-makeup-and-cosmetics-history.
11 Sava, Sanda. 2016. "A History of Make-Up & Fashion: 1900–1910—Sanda Sava | Make-Up Artist." Sanda Sava | Make-Up Artist. Accessed September 30, 2019. https://sandasava.com/beauty-style/a-history-of-make-up-fashion-1900-1910/.

Geoffrey Jones[12] adds:

> Television also proved a medium that new entrants could use to challenge incumbents. During the late 1950s, Leonard Lavin used television advertising to grow the tiny Alberto-Culver hair care business into a significant national player. More recently, home shopping channels such as HSN and QVC have become important places to launch new brands. However, the impact of television was not limited to marketing. Color television drove innovation in makeup, which was subsequently diffused from actors to the wider public. And as the United States became a major source of television programming worldwide, it proved a major force for diffusing American ideals of lifestyle, fashion, and beauty worldwide.[13]

In the twentieth century makeup became more democratized and a tool for everybody to use. Helena Rubinstein amongst others like Estée Lauder, Elizabeth Arden, and Coco Chanel, were women who succeeded in the beauty industry

---

12 "The History of Beauty." 2010. HBS Working Knowledge. Accessed September 30, 2019. https://hbswk.hbs.edu/item/the-history-of-beauty.

13 Ibid.

by putting their ideas and images out there.[14] Helena Rubinstein was a firm supporter of women in their movement for equality, "which throughout the twentieth century meant not only fighting for their most basic rights, but also for the liberation of their bodies and image of beauty—first by freeing them from the shackles of corsets and then from the taboo of wearing makeup. Until the early 1920s cosmetics were only worn by prostitutes and actresses."[15]

Geoffrey Jones adds to that:

> As for decorative cosmetics, the story of lipstick is really interesting. While the use of lipstick, like many cosmetics products, reaches back far into human history, in the early twentieth century it was still a product associated with actresses and women of dubious morality. Thereafter the use and acceptability of lipstick expanded. There was technological innovation—the first metal lipstick container was invented in Connecticut in 1915, and the first screw-up lipstick appeared six years later. By the time the United States entered World War II in 1941, the government declared the production of lipstick

14 Fitoussi, Michèle, Bignold, Kate, and Ramakrishnan Iyer, Lakshmi. *Helena Rubinstein: The Woman Who Invented Beauty*. London, Great Britain: Gallic Books, 2013.

15 Ibid.

to be a wartime necessity, such was its impact on morale...ever-feuding Helena Rubinstein and Elizabeth Arden, who transformed beauty salons from places considered the moral equivalent of brothels to palaces of opulence and style. [16]

Helena Rubinstein was influential in creating beauty as we know it today: scientific, rigorous, and demanding, with an emphasis on moisturizing, protecting against harmful rays of the sun, massage, electricity, hydrotherapy, hygiene, diet, nutrition, physical exercise and surgery. Her point of view was, "beauty is anything but frivolous" and that it was "a new power," a means through which women could assert their independence. [17]

In my opinion, Helena Rubinstein had a lovely way of talking about the beauty industry. In its purest form, Rubinstein changed the global beauty industry for consumers forever by giving women the power to *feel* beautiful no matter what. Estée Lauder did so as well, with her famous quote "Every woman can be beautiful, and I will show you how."

16 "The History of Beauty." 2010. *HBS Working Knowledge.* Accessed September 30, 2019. https://hbswk.hbs.edu/item/the-history-of-beauty.

17 Fitoussi, Michèle, Bignold, Kate, and Ramakrishnan Iyer, Lakshmi. Helena Rubinstein: The Woman Who Invented Beauty London, Great Britain: Gallic Books, 2013.

For Rubinstein, "To want to charm or look your best are not signs of subservience if you know how to use them to your advantage."[18] She believed women must use their assets placed at their disposal if they are to conquer the world, or at least to make their place in it.

As Jeanne Chavez[19] says:

> Today, the popular look and feel is definitely in what we are seeing with surgical enhancements. Personally, I don't judge that at all. I don't think it's bad to want to alter how you look because it's in our nature to want to do so. What keeps us balanced is that most of the time we can see two parallel tracks. One on each extreme, one with more of an "altered" look and another on the more "natural" look and then of course everything in between.

I think it is unfair that many people are shamed for wanting to alter or enhance something they do not *feel* confident about. Now with so much innovation and science going on in the beauty industry, searching for better ingredients and

---

18 Ibid.

19 Jeanne Chavez is the President and co-founder of the beauty brands, Smith & Cult, and the co-founder of Hard Candy. She has had a decades-long career in beauty, starting off at Orlane Institute to luxury brand La Prairie before ending up at her current position.

more potent formulas, we as consumers have a lot more to choose from when it comes to beauty routines, treatments, and enhancements.

A renowned professional in the medical aesthetic industry who has requested to remain anonymous mentioned that years ago the medical aspect of beauty was not too famous. Now, it is the main focus of the business, meaning this is a peak moment to experiment with all aspects of beauty—from the most inner and foundational to the outermost and physical aspects of beauty.

We have now reached a point where the majority of the world's population lives above the poverty line, violence is at an all-time low, and the overall happiness index is at a peak. Because fewer people spend their days worrying about survival, we have more time for leisure and the pursuit of pleasure, including the cultivation of our well-being. Having more time to invest in personal capital and image, the 445-billion-dollar beauty industry will become of even greater relevance going forward.

WHERE IS BEAUTY FOUND?

Beauty is the emotional intensity of being mesmerized by someone, an unexplainable attraction and curiosity to them. It is a reminder of the unexplainable nature of life itself.

This does not necessarily mean someone is sexually attractive or physically symmetrical. Rather, it refers to someone who strikes you, and not only by their appearance.

However, I don't think outer beauty should be neglected, as it is also a component of how an individual's beauty is perceived. The problem is there has been a capitalization on external beauty in society, which has caused more people's mental health to be negatively affected by reasons related to what it means to be beautiful.

The important connection to be aware of is that outer beauty heavily depends on your physical internal health and mental health. A dominant inner beauty can drastically enhance your physical outer beauty. It can give you the confidence and the extra "umph" you need to make sure you are being the best version of yourself—at home, at work, and anywhere else you may be.

Feeling proud of yourself, of the way you look, of your identity, of your features, of your color, of your ethnicity, of your culture, is what feeling beautiful is all about.

It all comes down to confidence.

Outer appearance, although I would love to say does not matter to the component of beauty, does play a role. However, it is only a fraction of the equation.

In this technology-suffocated era, it is crucial for people to own their confidence, to practice self-love, and to focus on inner beauty, so the technology can be used as a tool of knowledge and exposure, rather than one that hampers authenticity from flourishing.

Owning your beauty, your look, your confidence, your thoughts, your actions, and your identity makes you radiate. A confident and genuine smile, helping an elderly person cross the road, telling a story with passion, expressing genuine interest, and a look that shows you are present are just a few examples. It is an important human right to be able to live a life where each day you *feel* confident and worthy so you can explore causes beyond yourself.

NO BETTER COSMETIC

Bisila Bokoko[20] is not only a successful role model for our society, who positively impacts everything she touches, but she is also one of the most vibrant, splendid, and passionate women I have ever met. She is BEAUTIFUL.

---

20 Bisila Bokoko is the founder and CEO of BBES, a business development agency in New York that represents and promotes international market brands. She has inspired thousands of people and organizations around the world through conferences in which she has motivated others to pursue dreams, think big, and talk about empowerment, entrepreneurship, geopolitics, and personal branding.

Contagiously beautiful. However, she once felt ugly and unworthy until she changed her life by changing her perception of herself.

Now, Bisila's motto for life is "Smiling is my lifestyle."

> I think beauty is in the eyes of the beholder, and the perception of beauty is coming from the outside. But if you work on your inner beauty, it will have an effect on how your external beauty is perceived. Beauty is your radiance. You cannot control your genes, but you can control your walk-in life. Other factors can also make you more beautiful—your style, your communication with society, and most importantly, your smile.
>
> —BISILA BOKOKO

"There is no better cosmetic than a nice smile."

—BISILA BOKOKO

I do agree with Bisila. The sexiest, most attractive, and beautiful cosmetic for all is a confident smile. It makes your beauty radiate—your passions, thoughts, ideas, humor, charisma, compassion, behavior, respect, empathy, love, etc... —to everyone around you.

How individuals choose to emanate their own inner beauty and energy varies. Some people don't wear any makeup, which is fantastic. Others want to put on some red lipstick and a thick layer of mascara, which is just as amazing. It's completely up to the individual. Whatever makes you *feel* beautiful and confident is what you should do.

After all, your external beauty mainly serves as the vehicle to transmit your true inner beauty.

Bisila says, "Beauty is the key to success in people. However, this beauty does not depend on how attractive you are physically. Think *Game of Thrones*. The attractive antagonists are incredibly disliked. Then think Mother Teresa. Through the actions she has performed, anyone would perceive her as a beautiful woman, regardless of her appearance."

I want to share a deeply personal story that Bisila told me in our time together that embodies the power of *feeling* beautiful. Bisila shared with me how hard it was for her to grow up in a country like Spain, where very few people looked like her. She went to a school that was predominantly white, and as you may know, little kids can be mean. Kids would tell her she couldn't sit with them because she didn't look like them. Some even made despicable comments like, "You are dark, so you are ugly."

Growing up in an environment like this made her feel as though she wasn't beautiful. Because the perception of beauty of the people she was surrounded by was not one that looked like her, she thought she would never be regarded as beautiful. As she got older, she gained weight, which made her feel more self-conscious and less beautiful.

After some time, however, Bisila began to change her perception of beauty.

> I realized we are our first and worst critic, so decided I needed to see myself as beautiful. Technology actually helped me deal with my emotions, as I was seeing a growing democratization in beauty spread on digital platforms. So, I began to work with photographers who would take pictures of me to celebrate my beauty. I became the image of my own brand and I began to feel more confident in myself the more I did this. Before, even black models and other ethnic models were still the ones who looked whitewashed. But with more exposure to different looks and features, I got the courage to start modeling for my brands.

Inner beauty can change your outer beauty as you heal and strengthen your self-confidence.

Mental and physical health is important to feel beautiful too. In my opinion, social media is a tool that can help us feel more beautiful; it can help us understand that beauty exists in all types of people.

Bisila became confident in herself through caring for her inner beauty and letting it shine through. Once she started rewiring how she thought about her own beauty and fully believing she was beautiful, her physical appearance started to change. Crazy how the mind and body connection works. She lost a lot of weight, and her external beauty began to work in her favor because she felt good and was happy with herself. It is a ripple effect. Once you choose to change how you perceive yourself, everything around you begins to align with your inner beauty.

The first step for Bisila was believing she was beautiful.

When I was with her, her presence made me feel so warm and motivated, it was almost magical. It is clear from a distance that this woman radiates her inner beauty through her outer beauty the moment you look at her. She almost makes it impossible for you not to believe she is an inspiring beacon of beauty.

Feeling *beautiful trumps your need for physical appearance validation, every time.*

When you *feel* beautiful, you can better express your passions, your curiosities in life, what motivates you, and all that jazz. This allows you to communicate a part of your inner beauty that no one can take from you—the beauty that makes you, you.

Focus on seeing yourself as beautiful because if you don't *feel* beautiful, you cannot expect anyone else around you to see you as such. And remember, nothing is more captivating than a confident smile.

REASSESS WHAT BEAUTY MEANS TO YOU

With all the picture-perfect social media influencers, celebrities, and models, we are bombarded with images of what we "should" look like. A lot of us also place our self-worth on the amount of likes we get on a certain post. We see "likes" as validation from society. But, thankfully, the beauty industry is changing for the better.

Buzzwords like *anti-aging* are becoming more and more frowned upon while skin health and ingredient awareness are becoming more prominent. There is a visible shift in the course of the beauty industry toward a more inclusive direction. For instance, incorporating all skin-tones and genders is now a significant part of the beauty conversation. We are experiencing a time when the pressure to subscribe to a standard of beauty is becoming less appealing.

Only when we have a clear mind and see things from the perspective that beauty comes from the inside out will we foster a relationship with ourselves and with the beauty industry that allows us to appreciate our own power of *feeling* beautiful.

If we focus on beauty as empowerment, the beauty industry will no longer capitalize on people's insecurities and will shift to making individuals feel like the best version of themselves.

CHAPTER 2

YOUR PERCEPTION OF BEAUTY

———

Beauty is an ambiguous and subjective concept that each person sees in their own way.

Distracted by the cycle of our everyday routines, we often do not take the time to ask ourselves:

What is my perception of beauty?

Who do I see as beautiful?

My mother, father, grandmother, sibling, cousin, best friend, acquaintance, colleague, influencer, model, actress... Who?

Instead of setting guidelines of who we view as beautiful and why, we tend to take the easy way out and subscribe to standards of beauty that society imposes upon us. We tend to conclude that beauty is a set of certain parameters we must abide by.

I ask myself this question all the time: *What is MY perception of beauty?*

I realize that the people I find most beautiful are the ones who have charm. I mean, of course many women and men are genetically gifted with being objectively attractive. That is something no one can deny. Yet, just because they are physically attractive does not mean they are beautiful.

BEAUTY DOES NOT EQUAL SEX APPEAL

To me, beauty is something that makes you want to smile when you look at someone.

It's largely dependent on an individual's kindness, sincerity, sympathy, compassion, endearing mannerisms, and a look— their Signature Feature as Dr. Shamban calls it.[21]

---

21 Dr. Ava Shamban is the owner and director of two branded practices— AVA MD, her full-service Dermatology clinics in Santa Monica, Beverly Hills, and new concept SKINFIVE in West LA/Century City and Pacific Palisades. She is a renowned board-certified dermatologist, true skin visionary, clinician, author, anti-aging expert, prejuvenation proponent, and now co-host on The GIST Show.

Beauty lies in how we perceive ourselves and the people who surround us.

Beauty is some sort of magic, like a sixth sense. When you are with someone and you feel they are present, they are well with themselves, they are radiant, they are healthy, and they are connected. Our body is the vehicle that allows us to express that beauty.

Although your internal mindset and feeling affects your outer beauty significantly, enhancing your external beauty can also affect the way you feel internally. This is a completely normal scenario and nothing of which to be ashamed.

In fact, if done purposefully and for the right reasons, enhancing our beauty becomes part of taking care of and loving ourselves.

Think about your body and your external beauty as a car. Imagine you have a beautiful expensive car, let's say a Porsche, but you have nowhere to go and no place to be. While this vehicle is a luxurious and attractive car to have, it's not serving any purpose. This is like people who are objectively attractive and may have sex appeal but have little to offer on the inside. They might be unhealthy, mentally unstable, or have some aspect of their personality that simply does not appeal to you. Now let's say you have a Mazda, but you have places to go, people to see, and things to do. While this car is not as dressy on the outside as a Porsche Panamera, it still serves the purpose of transportation, not to mention it is less expensive to maintain, and it gets you to your destination.

Ultimately, this is to say that your physical beauty, the beauty people most often think and obsess about, is only your vehicle. Although the vehicle is important because it's the channel by which you radiate your inner beauty, it is more important to cultivate your inner beauty. If you don't, and you have nothing to offer, it will be hard to keep others captivated.

You possess the power of owning your own internal beauty to radiate out. You are in control of whether people see you as beautiful or not.

Beauty, especially beauty in human beings, is an intuitive emotion that consists of an interaction of delightful emotions and pleasure with one's presence.

IS BEAUTY IN THE EYE OF
THE BEHOLDER? NOT EXACTLY

"You know how beauty lies in the eyes of the beholder? Well, I disagree. It lies in your eyes. Who is beholding you? A guy said beauty is in the eyes of the beholder because beauty was only reserved to women before," said Priyanka Chopra Jonas[22] at BeautyCon LA 2019.[23]

Priyanka has a point. Although the verbatim form of the phrase was first coined by Margaret Wolfe Hungerford, an Irish novelist of the late nineteenth century, this saying first appeared in the third century BC in Greek and then was used by the English dramatist John Lyly in *Euphues and His England* in the late sixteenth century in the following format:

"...*as neere is Fancie to Beautie, as the pricke to the Rose, as the stalke to the rynde, as the earth to the roote.*"[24]

Priyanka continued by saying:

Don't get me wrong. It is fine to like someone appreciating you. It's fine to have a guy or a girl or whomever it may be telling you that you are

22 Priyanka Chopra Jonas is an Indian actress, model, singer, and film producer who began her fame when she won the Miss World 2000 pageant.

23 BeautyCon LA is a beauty festival that brings the best of the industry together for two days at the Los Angeles Convention Center.

24 Martin, Gary. 2019. "'Beauty Is In The Eye Of The Beholder'—The Meaning And Origin Of This Phrase." https://www.phrases.org.uk/meanings/beauty-is-in-the-eye-of-the-beholder.html.

beautiful, and this makes you feel good and feel yourself. All of that is fine but this is not where your validation should be coming from. This external affirmation is just a bonus. Your validation should be coming from your achievements, what you are up to, and your self-love.

We all have bad days when we feel like s***, and that is completely normal. With the advent of social media platforms, we often have a notion that we must look like we live a perfect life and always look fantastic. In reality, part of *feeling* beautiful is appreciating yourself in the hard days when everything seems to be going wrong and then on great days when you wonder how life can be so spectacular.

None of us are perfect! Not even the people who seem like they are. I, myself, have a struggle with assimilating this concept completely. Many years of ballet trained me to always strive for perfection. However, this does not translate to real life. I work on reminding myself about this time and again.

Although I have gotten a lot better at accepting it, something that has helped me when I catch myself trying to strive for perfection is reminding myself that "perfection is the enemy of great."

Focus on being great for yourself and not perfect for others.

As Priyanka said at BeautyCon LA, "Make sure you are not living life through someone else or through society's validation."

The most important takeaway about Priyanka's talk is that the perception of beauty is how you let others perceive yourself. It's not the other way around.

Essentially, the eye of the beholder only has as much power as you emanate. Within each of us lies the most powerful of all beauty. If we let that inner beauty radiate outward, it is impossible for the beholder not to see it.

Some people may agree with the saying "Beauty is in the eye of the beholder" because, of course, beauty is subjective… Right? Well, I hope you can now see that this statement is not entirely true. Beauty is in your power first, and only then, the beholder comes into play.

It all stems from you feeling it yourself. As Bisila[25] said, "Even a burn victim can be the most beautiful individual in the world."

---

25 Bisila Bokoko is the founder and CEO of BBES, a business development agency in New York that represents and promotes international market brands. She has inspired thousands of people and organizations around the world through conferences in which she has motivated others to pursue dreams, think big, and talk about empowerment, entrepreneurship, geopolitics, and personal branding.

TESTIMONIALS FROM THOSE WHO
WORK IN THE INDUSTRY

"Even when I was working in beauty companies where our main job was to work on enhancing people's physical appearance, we still believed we were enabling people, men and women, to look beautiful and feel beautiful, so their inner beauty could reflect outward."

—HEAD OF THE GREATER CHINA BEAUTY BUSINESS
AT A LEADING MULTINATIONAL CORPORATION.[26]

We tend to believe the people working in the industry think beauty is strictly an external factor. However, this is far from the truth. After speaking to sixty plus professionals, I have realized quite the opposite. Brands are beginning to convey what they truly believe—that external beauty cannot make you beautiful. It can only enhance your inner beauty.

Of all the questions I asked professionals, without a doubt, the question, "Can you define your own perception of beauty?" always caused a pause.

This was the case, regardless how high up the professional was in a company or the number of years they had been in

---

26 This industry professional wishes to keep personal and company information anonymous.

the industry. Some even confessed to me they had not ever put their own perception of beauty into words. It was simply something that just was.

Why don't you think about it for a moment?

What is YOUR personal definition of the perception of beauty? Hard, right?

Is it some type of physical tangible component of someone's appearance? Or, is it something that comes from a deeper level of human understanding?

This rethinking of beauty may allow our society and the industry to reach their maximum potential in terms of the way we consume beauty and the transparency and authenticity in the presentation of beauty. It is a step closer to a win-win scenario, for both businesses and consumers. It seems as if nowadays, most businesses are based on a one-sided win.

WHAT DO THEY ACTUALLY THINK?

Professionals' perception of beauty can help us understand the gap that exists between what we think the beauty industry is trying to impose on our society and what ideas are actually being pushed from the people who lead the industry themselves.

I strongly believe the industry is going in a positive direction in conveying a more inclusive, honest, representative and authentic beauty standard; therefore, eliminating the concept of a fixed universal standard. As the professionals will tell you below, you need to believe in yourself and your own beauty.

Head of the Greater China beauty business at a leading multinational corporation:[27]

> Personally, I am a total believer of inside out beauty. A confident smile is how beauty best comes out. I have always thought this. Of course, as I have gotten older, I realize that beauty can come with wisdom, and wisdom comes from unique experiences. The more you know yourself, the more you are comfortable in your own skin, like Olay's motto used to be "Love the skin you're in." Ultimately, beauty is to be yourself and to love yourself. Particularly when talking about the amount of globalization, the unique identity of an individual is vital to their beauty.

Head of EMEA beauty business at a leading multinational corporation:[28]

---

27 This industry professional wishes to keep personal and company information anonymous.
28 This industry professional wishes to keep personal and company information anonymous.

Beauty is a lot about energy, and every time I think a person is beautiful, I think the energy they are transmitting is beautiful. Beauty is when you get a great feeling in their presence. And based on that, you can think someone is beautiful. Even their imperfections can be a perfection. It is incredible how much someone's beauty can change in the course of a conversation. I am sure you have definitely had the experience of meeting someone you thought was incredibly attractive from afar, then got to meet them a little closer and realized their self-confidence and their way of caring for themselves made them less attractive than they were before. But there's also that person I'm sure you have also met that didn't exactly look so aesthetically proportionate or so harmonious to the eye from afar, yet they had the most powerful presence and self-confidence that immediately made you see the person as beautiful.

Ewelina Aiossa:[29]

Beauty is a combination of perceived qualities—such as physical appearance, features, shape, proportions—and intangible assets—such as personality traits, attitude,

---

29 Ewelina Aiossa is the Assistant Vice President of Marketing at SkinCeuticals, L'Oreal. She serves on UBM—Dermatology Times Industry Council and SkinCeuticals (SC) Leadership Team panel. She has a strong knowledge of the aesthetic business, professional channel, products, and ingredients.

mindset. The more graceful, charming, authentic, confident, and positive I find a person to be, the more beautiful they are to me, regardless if they meet the physical beauty standard criteria established by our society. I am personally drawn to people with a radiant soul and positive outlook who embrace their uniqueness and individuality (often imperfect by definition). I happen to find them to be more attractive physically—as their inner beauty radiates outward. It is scientifically proven that people who practice gratitude, stay true to their values, and are optimistic—have less "angry" expression lines and their skin radiates a happy and healthy glow while the ones with "heavy hearts" and a negative mindset have accentuated wrinkles, which our society finds less aesthetically appealing.

Dr. Ava Shamban:[30]

I believe everybody has a unique look to them, which is very important because if you are in a large community, why would you want to look like somebody else? If you did, people wouldn't remember you. The

---

30 Dr. Ava Shamban is the owner and director of two branded practices—AVA MD, her full-service Dermatology clinics in Santa Monica, Beverly Hills and new concept SKINFIVE in West LA/Century City and Pacific Palisades. She is a renowned board-certified dermatologist, true skin visionary, clinician, author, anti-aging expert, prejuvenation proponent, and now co-host on The GIST Show.

most important thing about beauty is to be memo-rable. We know this because of icon beauty. When we look at the older generation of signature beauty icons, they certainly didn't enhance themselves in the way people are enhancing themselves now.

Anastasia Soare:[31]

Beauty is about balance and proportion—not per-fection. This is the cornerstone with which Anas-tasia Beverly Hills was built. The eye is trained to recognize balance, and by using cosmetics and the right tools, it's possible to create greater harmony. I believe women should be able to see beauty as a source of empowerment. It's not about covering up or changing completely. It's about embracing your-self. It has the capability of reflecting confidence and security in that sense of self. And ultimately, what makes you feel powerful is what makes you most beautiful.

---

31 Anastasia Soare is the founder, CEO, and driving force behind Anastasia Beverly Hills—one of the fastest-growing brands in the beauty industry. In 1990, she introduced a new brow shaping technique to clients—later patented as the Golden Ratio Eyebrow Shaping Method—that has gone on to become a modern beauty essential. Anastasia is a beauty pioneer and powerhouse.

Dr. John Martin:[32]

> Beauty is very much determined by our culture, and many things combine to create "beauty." A person who is considered beautiful will appear healthy and fit. We look for facial symmetry and balance. The eyes are usually the most important feature for appearing attractive, so that is where I like to focus first. One of the most important things in cosmetic surgery is to make the person appear natural. If overdone or unnatural appearing, the person will often appear less attractive and more aged. People who are happy and confident (and smile) will also appear more beautiful.

The Head of LATAM at a leading multinational beauty company:[33]

> Beauty is individual. It is based on an individual bringing forward the features they want to celebrate. Beauty is about bringing out who you are. I like to think of beauty as a form of self-expression that is fluid between gender and ethnicities. When I think of beauty, even working at a color cosmetics company, I think of it not

---

32 Dr. John Martin is a Harvard-educated Medical Doctor who specializes in Facial Cosmetic Surgery as well as other non-surgical treatment for vascular and pigment problems as well as skin rejuvenation. Dr. Martin has been featured in *The Doctors, The Dr. Oz Show, Dr. Phil,* and *Anderson Cooper 360°.*

33 This industry professional wishes to keep personal and company information anonymous.

as top-down concept. No one should be telling you what beauty should look like. Rather you should be showing yourself and society what beauty can look like.

Jacinda Heintz:[34]

To me, beauty is a form of self-expression. It's the way you take care of yourself, the way you apply makeup, or the way you choose to wear nothing at all. These are all an extension of one's person and the way they desire to be perceived. One is most beautiful when they feel true to themselves, regardless of the standards set forth by the media or society. Whether it be a full face of makeup or an entirely bare face, I think the definition of beauty is unique to each individual.

Klara Chrzuszcz:[35]

Beauty is a broad term. It's not only superficial, but it's how someone feels and what they radiate. I do my

---

34 Jacinda Heintz is an Influencer Marketing Coordinator at Kendo Brands, Inc. She leverages her social media and marketing expertise to create socially driven partnerships that are mutually beneficial for both the brand and the influencer.

35 Klara Chrzuszcz is a Medical Skin care Aesthetician, Clinical Skin care Expert, and the owner of Klara Beauty Lab. Klara is an educator in Europe for neurotoxin application as well as dermal fillers for the face and body, and she travels to teach on a yearly basis. Her approach involves delving into clients' lifestyles, diets, stress levels, etc. which allows her to create a one-of-a-kind experience.

best to instill beauty and confidence in my clients, and seeing how they feel with their results is incredible. They leave my consultation with a different frequency than they came in with. To me, that is beauty. Beauty comes from within and I work with my patients to not only give them beautiful skin but to bring their inner beauty to the surface. Beauty is not only about looking good, but it's most importantly about feeling good.

Clémence von Mueffling:[36]

Beauty is not about looking like someone else or looking younger, but it's about looking and feeling like the best version of yourself. Make the most of what you were born with. I think that's really a positive perception of beauty because we must accept ourselves and use that to become the best version of who we can be. One of my favorite quotes from my book, *Ageless Beauty the French Way*, is from a very famous French writer who passed away just a few months ago, Jean D'Ormesson, *Guide des Égarés*,[37] "Beauty is pure magic that transforms the nature of existence."

---

36 Clémence von Mueffling is the Founder and Editor of Beauty and Well-Being (BWB), which brings a fresh aesthetic to the beauty and well-being media. She is also the author of *Ageless Beauty the French Way*, a luxurious, entertaining, unparalleled guide to every French beauty secret for all women.

37 Ormesson, Jean d'. *Guide des égarés* Paris: Gallimard, 2016.

Susana Martinez Vidal:[38]

I am convinced that beauty comes down to one's identity, personality, and style. As I wrote in my Instagram post: "Overestimating perfection and equating it to beauty is a mistake. It is your 'defects' or 'imperfections' that make you unique and give you your identity." Frida Kahlo is a great example of this; she owned her identity and her sticking eyebrow look. Sometimes that can be the most beautiful thing about a person. Beauty in the end is an intangible concept formed by many components, many of which are not external.

Roya Pourshalchi:[39]

Beauty is such a tough concept; for each one of us there's a cultural understanding of beauty, which affects how a person perceives themselves as beautiful.

---

38 Susana Martinez Vidal is a journalist and author, founder of *Ragazza* magazine, which catapulted her to becoming the youngest director of any edition of *Elle* in the world. After seeing the first exhibit of Frida Kahlo's clothing at the Casa Azul in 2012, she was inspired to write her first book, *Frida Kahlo: Fashion as the Art of Being*, recommended by *The New York Times* and *Vanity Fair* UK—most important magazines in more than twenty countries.

39 Roya Pourshalchi is a dedicated yoga teacher, Ayurveda consultant at Kilona Shop, and Marma bodywork therapist. Roya currently sees clients privately and hosts group classes and workshops in New York City. She is Yoga Alliance RYT-200 certified, trained in 100 HR Ayurveda Foundations and 100 HR Marma Therapy.

To me, beauty is an act of being. It's an act of being yourself in a way that brings joy into your life and is supportive of who you are. So being beautiful is not just about beautiful eyes or beautiful skin. It's about what you choose to invite into your life.

Chinwe Esimai:[40]

I think beauty is very subjective. When people talk about beauty, they often think about the physical. What do you see? And do you like what you see? But I strongly believe beauty comes from the inside out. Regardless of what is happening physically, if there is that projection, if there's a certain energy and confidence coming from the inside, you are influencing what you project and how people perceive what you project. Beauty is about really embracing who and what you and what you transmit out into the world.

Arden Martin:[41]

---

40 Chinwe Esimai is the Managing Director and Chief Anti-Bribery Officer at Citigroup, Inc. She is also an award-winning lawyer, author, and speaker who is passionate about inspiring generations of immigrant women leaders.

41 Arden Martin is a teacher of Vedic Meditation and co-founder of The Spring Meditation Studio in New York City. She cares deeply about bringing more transparency to the US personal care industry and works with Beautycounter to educate people about what "clean beauty" really means.

There is a huge push with the "glow" right now. Everyone wants glowing skin, and there is a reason for that. Glowing skin implies inner beauty as well as outer beauty to me. When you glow, you radiate energy from a place of a happy mental state and a healthy physical body. To me beauty is all about supporting your well-being from the inside out and from the outside in. Meditation has been the most transformative component of inner beauty for me as it has considerably boosted my confidence. After I started feeling good about myself, everyone started telling me I looked beautiful. It really all comes down to your stress and mental state, rather than your physical appearance.

Tyle Mahoney:[42]

"My perception of beauty is a subtle, natural, and sometimes understated one. I think you can shine your beauty and enhance the way you shine it, but tampering with it can take away from your beauty. I would never want to change what we were given because that is beauty—to be as we are."

---

42 Tyle Mahoney is an expert colorist with more than fifteen years of experience at MèCHE salon. Clients depend on him not only for his skill when it comes to creating the perfect color, but also for his ability to make his creations last. Considering lifestyle as well as the elements, Tyle tailors his methods to ensure fade-resistant color and shine. He works hand in hand with Tracey Cunningham.

Dr. Jouhayna Alouie:[43]

"Beauty is a unique and harmonious interaction between its elements. These elements include physical appearance, body language, expressive language, positive emotions, good health, intellectual reserve, and confidence. The way these elements interact together at different stages of life results in a balanced state of beauty that is unique and dynamic."

Greater China Vice President of one of the world's leading beauty manufacturing and marketing multinational companies:[44] "To me, beauty is about confidence and how you see yourself. The most important attributes of beauty are whether or not a person is happy and confident with themselves."

Yolanda Sacristán:[45] "For me beauty has a lot to do with the message a person transmits of themselves: attitude, empathy,

---

43 Dr. Jouhayna Alouie is a well-known esthetician in Beirut, Paris, and Riyadh, who has been working in the field since the mid-seventies. She specializes in corrective work, permanent makeup, and enhancement facial treatments. In the past, she has worked closely with Miss France and many Arab celebrities.

44 This industry professional wishes to keep personal and company information anonymous.

45 Yolanda Sactristán is the General Director of TheBeautyNewsroom. com and the former Editor-in-Chief of renowned publications: *Vogue* (2001-2017) and *Harper's Bazaar* (2017-2019). Yolanda is a skilled journalist with a passion for fashion, beauty, and luxury. She is always determined to produce compelling stories.

self-esteem, smile... in short, aspects that have to do with the personality and the projection of that personality."

Nayera Senane:[46] "I would say beauty is when people look natural. I believe everyone is beautiful in their own way and I like to enhance what they already have."

Jeanne Chavez:[47] "Basically, I think beauty can be shaped by what's happening in your life. It's not about how you look; it's really about how you feel."

French Montana:[48] "Beauty has to come from the inside, and you feel it when it comes from here (points to the heart). For me to think someone is beautiful, I need to feel it in their energy. You cannot lie about energy. If you know how to read energy, you can read beauty."

---

46 Nayera Senane is a Diamond Allergan Injector, Botox and dermal filler expert. She currently holds a wide client base including celebrities and models. Although based in Los Angeles, she travels regularly to the East Coast to see clients.

47 Jeanne Chavez is the President and co-founder of the beauty brands, Smith & Cult, and the co-founder of Hard Candy. She has had a decades-long career in beauty, starting off at Orlane Institute to luxury brand La Prairie before ending up at her current position.

48 French Montana is a Moroccan rapper who moved to the US at the age of thirteen. Now he is the founder and CEO Cocaine City Records.

Dr. Barbara Sturm:[49] "I think beauty is in people who are extremely friendly, kind, sweet, loving and giving. It's about how you radiate. I like to see beauty as something that has to do with your soul."

HOW DIFFERENT ARE THESE PERCEPTIONS REALLY?

These definitions of perceptions of beauty aren't all too different. How interesting, right?

We all invest so much time, energy, and money into *looking* beautiful on the outside, yet all the people working in the beauty industry agree that beauty comes from within.

Society has convinced us that we need to subscribe to a certain standard if we want to be beautiful. The argument can be made that this concept has been the driving force of revenue for beauty brands. However, if this is the case, I believe a lot more revenue can be made if the beauty industry incorporates more of the opinions of beauty shared by the professionals above. Here is a beauty where uniqueness

---

49 Dr. Barbara Sturm is the founder and CEO of Dr. Barbara Sturm Molecular Cosmetics. She is a German aesthetics doctor, widely renowned for her anti-inflammatory philosophy and her non-surgical anti-aging skin treatments. Dr. Sturm translated science from her clinical research and orthopedic practice into the field of aesthetics and has been a success ever since.

and authenticity are celebrated, where products can enhance inner beauty rather than pressure everyone to look the same.

In my opinion, the beauty industry is taking strides in the correct direction to push for this message of beauty. But for the time being, I hope these snippets will hold you over and transform how you think about beauty.

PERCEPTION OF BEAUTY FROM THE REGIONAL PERSPECTIVE

Although many beauty professionals around the world have similar perspectives on beauty, we must also consider cultural nuances. Around the world different cultures consider different features or ways of carrying oneself more beautiful than others.

To expose you to some of these distinctions, below are some of the key takeaways that professionals shared in regard to varying ideas on regional beauty around the world.

The Greater China Vice President of one of the world's leading beauty manufacturing and marketing multinational companies:[50]

---

50 This industry professional wishes to keep personal and company information anonymous.

With regards to skin brightening, there is an ancient Asian saying, "The fairness of your skin can hide flaws in your skin." In Asia, beauty is centered around having light and bright skin. Whitening skin care started with Japanese brands and from the 1980s and there has been little to no change in this mindset. It has only changed from focusing on superficially white skin to fair skin instead. Further, in Asian languages, there are different sayings to describe what beautiful skin must look like. The sayings range from skin that resembles the surface of a boiled-egg, to porcelain, to one that resembles the outside of Mochi ice cream— white-matte flawless skin.

Beauty lingo has slowly evolved from white skin to healthy, radiant, and translucent skin. To finish off, the Asian beauty product user can spend thirty to forty minutes on their twelve-step skin care morning and night routine because in Asia, beauty predominantly starts from the skin. Therefore, the skin care market is much bigger market than the color cosmetics one.

The Head of Greater China beauty business at a leading multinational corporation:[51]

---

51 This industry professional wishes to keep personal and company information anonymous.

In Asia, beauty is primarily about the whitening of the skin. Whitening is an important part of the culture because fair skin means status. There has been an evolvement with Asian beauty and it seems like the skin care and color cosmetics paths are crossing. The explosion of color cosmetics seems to be taking over the youth, not only as a form of beauty but as a form of expression. Over and beyond, the Generation Z and millennials are starting to express their identity through makeup.

Marie Englesson:[52]

Growing up in Sweden there is a lot of a natural inspiration, and it is considered beautiful to look natural. As such, for me beauty is looking natural and fresh, and feeling comfortable. When I started looking at beauty in Africa, I felt like the beauty industry focused on a beauty look that seemed "fake" and "imposed" on African people. It was obvious that the makeup they were using was not made for them. People did not know there was makeup to

52 Marie Englesson is now working as a retail and supply chain consultant in the East African region. Prior, she started up her own beauty retail and distribution business in Tanzania, called Atsoko. Starting from scratch, she developed a retail platform with seven stores and introduced twelve global beauty brands in the market. In early 2018, when she sold her business, Atsoko was ranked among the top one hundred medium-sized companies in Tanzania.

enhance their own natural beauty, and they didn't have to look like they were wearing a mask to look beautiful. This was mainly because they didn't have any products available to them to do so.

Chinwe Esimai:[53]

I was seventeen when my family moved to the US from Nigeria, in 1995. That was also the moment where I thought: "Wow, I look so different here." My features are so striking that there were moments when I was in the US that I wondered, "Do I really want to stick out THIS much?" A part of me coming into my own self-love was the ability to embrace myself in a place where people didn't necessarily look like me. I learned to embrace my identity. Now that I am raising an eleven-year-old daughter, I am able to emphasize to her that beauty is more than what you see on the surface. We need to be able to appreciate and be comfortable with different types of beauty. No matter where you go in the world, you may or may not stand out, but it's important to be comfortable being who you are.

---

53 Chinwe Esimai is the Managing Director and Chief Anti-Bribery Officer at Citigroup, Inc. She is also an award-winning lawyer, author, and speaker who is passionate about inspiring generations of immigrant women leaders.

Dr. Jouhayna Alouie:[54]

Beauty must be considered within cultural con-
texts. Each part of the world has its own unique culture and therefore its unique perception of beauty,
including Lebanon, where I am from. Having said
that, we need to keep in mind that as culture changes
around the world, the perception of beauty will follow. Globalization and technology/social media have
facilitated communications and exchanges among
people all over the world. There is no doubt that this
free flow of information has affected many aspects of
our lives including our perception of beauty, which
has become a broader and more inclusive one.

Yolanda Sacristán:[55]

As for Spanish society, it is possible that the universal social tendency to catalog everything leads
to a biased definition of beauty. This idea of beauty

---

54 Dr. Jouhayna Alouie is a well-known esthetician in Beirut, Paris,
    and Riyadh, who has been working in the field since the mid-
    seventies. She specializes in corrective work, permanent makeup,
    and enhancement facial treatments. In the past, she has worked
    closely with Miss France and many Arab celebrities.

55 Yolanda Sactristán is the General Director of TheBeautyNewsroom.
    com and the former Editor-in-Chief of renowned publications:
    Vogue (2001-2017) and *Harper's Bazaar* (2017-2019). Yolanda is a
    skilled journalist with a passion for fashion, beauty, and luxury.
    She is always determined to produce compelling stories.

is largely based on the analysis of physical beauty. Spanish societies are developed on a history of measurements and comparisons that start, in the case of beauty, by parameters imposed by fashions or trends of the moment. I refer to simple factors such as height, weight, shape of the face, color of hair or eyes, thickness of the lips and other elements that have to do with the external appearance of the person and the harmony of one's features with respect to these predefined parameters. This is how it has always worked. In this sense, I am pleased to see how the different societies are maturing in a desire to redefine beauty in a more complete, global, and holistic way, incorporating personality factors that were not evident nor were considered, until recent years.

Clémence von Mueffling:[56]

When I moved to the US from France about twelve years ago, I was given the opportunity to dive into the world of beauty in America. This allowed me to see the contrast between American and French standards of beauty. One of the main differences I realized is that

---

56 Clémence von Mueffling is the Founder and Editor of Beauty and Well-Being (BWB), which brings a fresh aesthetic to the beauty and well-being media. She is also the author of *Ageless Beauty the French Way*, a luxurious, entertaining, unparalleled guide to every French beauty secret for all women.

in France, women don't fight their age as much as they do in the US. The idea of beautiful skin is not about flawless skin but healthy skin in France. On the other hand, in the US there is a quest for flawless skin. I think sometimes when one's end goal is perfection, they can end up making some decisions that might not be the best for their skin's health, such as aggressive treatments.

I think French women see that we only have one skin and one face, and we must take care of it. Rather than focusing on removing their wrinkles and fine lines, they focus on cultivating a healthy and glowing skin. As I like to say, you have to treat the skin of your face like your favorite silk blouse.

The main difference is that French women settle with great skin and don't need perfectly flaw-less skin to be content. The process to get to this great skin is part of our culture. This is a routine a mother will teach her daughter in her teenage years. This culture of preventative skin care begins from a young age, which includes regimens such as double cleansing, using thermal water, applying the right moisturizer, etc. Your skin is the result of how you have been treating yourself in both the past and present. The quest for perfection is not only hard to attain but also frustrating. Aim for great instead.

Teresa De La Cierva:[57]

The Spanish in general use makeup in an emotional way to create an illusion in times of crisis for example. Spanish people in general have a lot of self-love. They rarely alter their features due to aesthetics, or if they do, usually it is due to a large insecurity or abnormality. In Spain I would say that the "natural look" is very well perceived.

Previously, the Spanish did not take care of their skin much, when it came to to sunbathing and tanning beds. It has always been part of the Spanish perception of beauty that someone who was tan looked more beautiful. Now, it is true that with the knowledge on the harmful causes of tanning, the Spanish are beginning to take care of their skin, especially when it comes to sun exposure and pollution, but they still have a long way to go. I think the era of influencers is also bringing a vision toward cosmetic treatments that are much more normalized than ever before in Spain, especially among the youth.

---

57   Teresa De La Cierva is an excellent journalist and communicator, working for ABC writing about beauty for almost her entire career. She started writing on paper and then created one of the first five blogs in the newspaper, called "La Polvera," which was about beauty. She is frequently featured speaking about beauty on Federico Jiménez Losantos' radio show on esRadio's Morning.

Head of EMEA beauty business at a leading multinational corporation:[58]

> In the Gulf countries, beauty is huge. These women are big consumers of high-quality makeup. The misconception that women in this region are not big beauty consumers because they cover themselves for religious reasons is false. They actually consume just as much as the average woman who does not cover herself. They wear makeup at home or in their intimacy.

Mi Anne Chan:[59]

> With social media, the beauty industry is in the process of democratizing. Trends that are born in Asia become large fads in the United States, and vice versa. However, what is "beautiful" can definitely change from place to place. For example, in contrast to the US, in Asia, there's still a huge onus put on being pale. Women in Asia also covet dewy skin, as seen in the "glass skin" trend in South Korea.

---

58 This industry professional wishes to keep personal and company information anonymous.

59 Mi Anne Chan is an Associate Producer and Staff Writer at Refinery29, a video director at Condé Nast entertainment, and a beauty influencer/ vlogger. She has been writing, editing, filming, and making tutorials on all things beauty related since the start of her career.

Marie Englesson:[60]

Living in Africa I have seen the focus on skin and
skin tone, and the link it has with beauty. Unfortunately, the fairer the skin, the more beautiful. While
there is a growing pride in being African and African
beauty, there is still very much a social hierarchy and
status derived from the complexion of one's skin. It
is also important to note that East and West African
beauty standards are worlds different. It is important
to keep pushing to find local models. Local beauty
is how beauty should be showcased.

Anne Booth Dayton:[61]

Through living in Asia and through my work at Christie's, I have witnessed the perception of beauty unfold
from different regions of the world. In Japan, for example, beauty is commonly found in the nape of the neck,
therefore the kimono collar is tilted far back and open

---

60 Marie Englesson is now working as a retail and supply chain
    consultant in the East African region. Prior, she started up her own
    beauty retail and distribution business in Tanzania, called Atsoko.
    Starting from scratch, she developed a retail platform with seven
    stores and introduced twelve global beauty brands in the market. In
    early 2018, when she sold her business, Atsoko was ranked among
    the top one hundred medium-sized companies in Tanzania.
61 Anne Booth Dayton is the Director of Institutional Advancement
    at El Museo del Barrio and previously was the Chief Operating
    Officer at Collectrium, a Christie's Company.

to expose the nape. The notion of beauty and sensual appeal is also reflected in mannerisms. For example, the way women walk is considered a type of erotic beauty. In Asia, this was the inspiration for foot binding to ensure tiny feet and the commensurate gait.

Jacinda Heintz:[62]

"An aspect of beauty that transcends all cultural nuances is the self-confidence and self-love one has for themselves. The power in beauty lies in self-expression and is unique to each person. It's truly all about showcasing what makes an individual feel most beautiful as themselves both internally and externally."

DO SOME CULTURES INHERENTLY *FEEL* MORE BEAUTIFUL THAN OTHERS?

1. In a society or culture where everyone looks just like one another, individuals may have a greater sense of belonging because people don't try to look like anyone else.

---

62 Jacinda Heintz is an Influencer Marketing Coordinator at Kendo Brands, Inc. She leverages her social media and marketing expertise to create socially driven partnerships that are mutually beneficial for both the brand and the influencer.

2. If a culture is taught from a young age to dress, walk, look, feel, and behave as though they are beautiful, people have a larger chance to inherently *feel* more beautiful.

As a Venezuelan woman, Jenny Villasana[63] shows one example of how the second can be true. She explains how in Venezuela a large emphasis is placed on *feeling* beautiful from a young age. I have numerous Venezuelan friends who have shared similar sentiments. As such, I found this anecdote both humorous and illuminating.

Jenny recounts:

> Miss Venezuela's beauty pageant TV program was one that nobody in the country could stop watching. No one. Everybody watched the TV program all year round. Every month of the year, we were soaking up the Misses in each region of Venezuela: Ms. Guarico, Ms. Federal District, ... and then the big day arrived once a year where everyone got beautiful to watch the finale of the Ms. Venezuela TV program in their own homes. I was twelve or thirteen years old, yet I still remember that we all dressed up and put makeup on to watch the finale. Although we were just watching

---

63 Jenny Villasana is a top certified Life Coach, Author of Children's books, and Radio Talk Show Host at *El Carrousel de tus Sueños / Cadena Azul* 1550 am.

the TV program we dressed up for ourselves, to feel as beautiful as the contestants; because as we were trained, one day we could be a Miss too.

"Strait back like a Miss Caramba! Have the look of a Miss! Walk like a Miss!" So, it was with moms, with teachers, with grandmothers. It was normal to be told this if you were a young girl growing up in Venezuela. Everyone had the resources went through etiquette academics. There was a famous one called Herman's Institute, where we didn't just go to be a Miss in the Miss Venezuela's TV program, but to also learn to be Miss—as for us it was important to act like a Miss at all times. It was part of our idio-syncrasy and our ideology as Venezuelan woman.

Beautiful women who had little resources presented themselves to the governor of their state many times to gain a sponsorship to enter the competition of Miss Venezuela. It was THAT important. The only thing they would have to be able to afford was the dress, but through their friends, family, or godpar-ents, somehow everyone always had someone they knew who would sponsor a dress for them.

You can talk to anyone in the world and I can tell you that the stereotype in Venezuela is one of two—petroleum and beautiful women. Not only because they were physically beautiful, but because many believed they were beautiful. Hence, others saw them as such.

Of course, there is a whole dark and negative side to all of this, creating an obsessive culture amongst women and what they were supposed to look and feel like. But there were also many incredible things about this culture, giving women like myself and many I know an inherent confidence in who we were. This feeling that we would always be beautiful no matter what happens in life is so ingrained in our upbringing that no one can take it from us. That is the power of the Venezuelan woman.

After reading the perceptions of professionals, we can come to the consensus that beauty is an art of living. The perception of human beauty comes first and foremost from within.

While we can always do things to enhance our external beauty—taking care of our skin and body, wearing makeup, living a mindful lifestyle, and more—it all begins with the way in which we perceive ourselves and how we feel.

PART II

WHAT WE PRACTICE

CHAPTER 3

SUBCONSCIOUSLY SUBSCRIBING TO TRENDS, BEHAVIORS AND EXPECTATIONS

———

It is not a negative attribute to subscribe to trends. It's only normal. However, it is important to analyze if these are trends we want to follow with intent. This way we can avoid any extra pressures that seem to tell us we are not enough.

It should be your choice to subscribe—a choice that makes you feel more you. Being a conscious participant in the industry and avoiding falling into the habit of subscribing to trends just because they are "in" with no internal reflection about how they make you feel is difficult. Yet, doing so will help you become more aware of yourself and what makes **you** *feel* good.

According to research conducted by Dove global on Dove's "Choose Beautiful" campaign surveying 6,400 women ages eighteen to sixty-four from five prominent cities around the world, the results were the following:[64]

- Only 4 percent of women around the world consider themselves beautiful.[65]
- Only 11 percent of girls globally are comfortable describing themselves as "beautiful."[66]
- 72 percent of girls feel tremendous pressure to be beautiful[67]
- 80 percent of women agree that every woman has something about her that is beautiful.[68]
- 54 percent of women globally agree they are their own worst beauty critics.[69]

To understand what might be propagating these numbers, let's look at what the industry is made up of and how we behave in relation to it.

---

64 2019. *Dove.Com*. Accessed October 4, 2019. https://www.dove.com/us/en/stories/about-dove/our-research.html.
65 Ibid.
66 Ibid.
67 Ibid.
68 Ibid.
69 Ibid.

WHAT THIS INDUSTRY IS MADE OF

The Head of LATAM at a leading multinational beauty company said to me:[70]

> Some people tend to think the world of beauty is easy and simple. You take a product out in the market, create some marketing campaigns, select a couple of models/influencers to promote it, give it a good brand name, and people buy it.

> Well, that is one way you look at it, but if you want to do it well, and you want to be the best at what you do in the industry, you need to understand the consumer, have cutting edge, breakthrough products that other brands don't offer, or you must tell the story of an untapped market. In order to nail all of this, you need to have done your research.

Conglomerates

The Chief Marketing Officer at a leading multinational beauty company said to me:[71]

---

70 This industry professional wishes to keep personal and company information anonymous.

71 This industry professional wishes to keep personal and company information anonymous.

Multinational companies and corporations like L'Oréal, Coty, Estée Lauder Companies, Procter & Gamble, Shiseido, etc. are now trying to portray their image of beauty as inclusive and diverse. They are achieving this by acquiring niche brands from all over the world that better represent people and their interests. This is enabling conglomerates to stay relevant in these times of rapid change in the industry. These big conglomerates not only need to acquire indie and niche brands to stay relevant and survive, but they must also adapt to the way other cultures perceive beauty more than ever before through their choice in the brands they add to their portfolios.

Inclusivity in the beauty standards of conglomerates are relatively new. As Anne Booth Dayton[72] noted, the beauty conglomerates did not have this approach in the past. Companies and brands went more by what she called "visual colonization," meaning that conglomerates implemented their standard of beauty in every country they entered.[73] Now, companies are steering away from this approach and achieving a more democratic perception of beauty for all consumers to feel identified and represented—not only in

---

72 Anne Booth Dayton is the Director of Institutional Advancement at El Museo del Barrio and previously was the Chief Operating Officer at Collectrium, a Christie's Company.

73 Ibid.

their perception of beauty, but also in their specific product consumption patterns and product usage behaviors.[74]

Indie Brands

Indie brands, companies that are independently owned and do not receive any corporately backed funding, work differently. Some examples of indie brands are Tammy Fender, Eminence, Kopari, and Mad Hippie, amongst many. These brands are seeing a lot of success from today's consumers because they cater directly to their needs and demands. For this reason, indie brands that have the potential are the biggest targets for conglomerates to acquire. Conglomerates can then can ensure that the perception of beauty they are communicating is as diversified and is covering as many bases of niche markets as they can all while keeping their core values.

I Call It Magic

Indie brands have given consumers the opportunity to use products that make them feel good and confident every day. Consumers don't purchase from a brand because the brand claims it has top products, but rather because consumers believe the brand truly cares about them, their interests, and their well-being.

---

74 Ibid.

The Head of Marketing LATAM at a leading multinational beauty company[75] gave me a great example of an experience they had when acquiring an indie brand for their conglomerate. The professional said:

> I have a lot of respect and compassion for the founder of a high-end Haircare Brand Y that we acquired some years back and tried to scale up. Our strategy at Multinational Company X that I was a part of at the time was to distribute a lower price tier of Haircare Band Y that would be available for mass consumption in retailers like Target and Walmart while also retaining a top tier more exclusive line in the portfolio.
>
> When certain high-end brands are acquired, tiering is a common, approach which allows for brand expansion via an accessible price point. With two levels of the business, one is available for mass consumption while the other, which retains and carries the image and maximum performance of the brand, is still sold in more select salons and retailers.
>
> Frankly, we focused too much on scaling and not enough on differentiated lineups for Hair Care Brand Y and we ended up having to shutter the entire operation.

---

75 This industry professional wishes to keep personal and company information anonymous.

Fortunately, the founder was able to independently recover his brand and is now expanding into different categories on his own terms, which was always his vision. The challenge is that brands often lose their aspirational image with expansion into mass markets and ultimately the original fanbase leaves the fold.

Many, not all, conglomerates' main goal is to acquire and scale without having incidents like these. They must respect and honor the consumer base and the values of a brand in order to have a diverse portfolio of beauty brands that maintain their equity for many generations.

The Head of Marketing LATAM at a leading multinational beauty company continued by saying:

> I think consumers have very high expectations of brands, especially within the realm of beauty. For this reason, we see the success of small niche beauty brands. There's this trend of beauty business leaders picking up the small niche brands in order to convey the feeling of a "small innovative and agile business," which can lend street credibility to these bigger and slower but well-funded conglomerates.

This *niche-beauty effect* is changing the industry drastically. This new trend is making products and brands have less competition amongst each other and allowing them to rely more on word of mouth and influencer marketing. These kinds of marketing have proven successful in enabling brands to reach people who before would have been deemed unreachable and get their products into the hands of the consumers in a more direct and efficient way than ever before.

According to the previously mentioned Head of Marketing LATAM, some multinationals have a more successful history of acquiring niche brands than others. By better, she means better at holding on to the values and story—the essence—of a brand. A great example of this is Estée Lauder. They are known to be a beauty house that nurtures the different creators and designers they acquire. Estée Lauder lets the companies protect their "essence" while providing the resources, supervision, and leadership from a big umbrella company that they need to grow.

Luxury Brands

Although the image of beauty is still toward inclusivity, there lies a specific look, feel, and story that luxury brands must reflect—their brand DNA. The maintenance of their foundational pillars take precedent over adapting to beauty trends of the moment. Luxury brands desire a fashion-forward and creative outlook for their beauty products and on the image of their brand. It's an aspirational feeling that consumers are looking for when they look into a luxury brand for anything beauty related, akin to what you would find in fashion. Therefore, no matter if a consumer in Asia, Europe, the Middle East, or Latin America desires a luxury product, they all gravitate toward these luxury brands such as Dior, Chanel, or Yves Saint Laurent for the same reason. They want the brand's specific look.

Oliver Lechére[76] explained that in Europe, when the economy crashed in 2008, luxury brands, especially in the fragrance and beauty business, had to face aggressive promotional activities from the wholesale distribution. These promotional activities, in certain ways, affected the exclusivity of luxury products. Since then, more people, especially younger people are more willing to invest in products of this caliber. This could very much have been caused by the promotional activities that happened about a decade ago, making consumers, especially millennials, more comfortable with the purchasing of luxury beauty products.

A Generation Z beauty connoisseur and university student and influencer from Hong Kong said to me,[77] "In Hong

---

76 Olivier Lechère is the General Director for Chanel Spain & Portugal in charge of the three divisions: Fashion, Fragrance & Beauty and Watches & Fine Jewelry in Madrid. He has dedicated these last twenty years to driving and growing the business by setting up two fashion flagship stores, boosting the fragrances and beauty division to number one in the Spanish market.

77 This person wishes to keep personal information anonymous.

Kong we teenagers are exposed to a variety of skin products, from affordable to luxury beauty products. As we grow older, we tend to 'step up our game,' meaning shifting from using affordable skin products to using luxury products like Chanel, YSL, Giorgio Armani, and all of those." This reinforces that younger generations are more comfortable with luxury products than any other generation before regardless of income.

GENERATIONS: CAN WE KEEP UP WITH THEM ALL?

The global beauty industry now has the most diversified consumer pool ever. Generation Z and millennials have been raised in the era of having a double life, IRL (in real life) and in digital life. Because of this, we have a huge shift in the demands of consumers.

Generation Z: Born 1997-Present
Millennials: Born 1981-1996
Generation X: Born 1965-1980
Baby Boomers: Born 1946-1964
Silent Generation: Born 1925-1945[78]

---

78 "New Guidelines Redefine Birth Years for Millennials, Gen-X, And 'Post-Millennials.'" 2018. *Mentalfloss.Com.* Accessed October 4 2019. http://mentalfloss.com/article/533632/new-guidelines-redefine-birth-years-millennials-gen-x-and-post-millennials.

Let's look at both millennials and Generation Z.

Millennials

Yolanda Sacristán[79] explained very eloquently the effect that the millennial generation is having on the beauty industry. She said:

> The millennial generation represents a challenge when attracting different markets and this stands in the case of beauty. In my opinion, this generation has different values, objectives, and priorities than those of the age groups that are currently in charge of organizations. Knowing their particularities is essential when developing productive and long-term relationships with brands and products. In this sense, the beauty market will have to understand and take into account some of its common features. For example, their need to be permanently connected to the internet; their egocentricity, understood by how they generate close relationships with their favorite brands and not

---

79 Yolanda Sactristán is the General Director of TheBeautyNewsroom.com and the former Editor-in-Chief of renowned publications: *Vogue* (2001-2017) and *Harper's Bazaar* (2017-2019). Yolanda is a skilled journalist with a passion for fashion, beauty, and luxury. She is always determined to produce compelling stories.

with any brand; their need to prioritize the care of the environment and sustainability; their search for flexibility and constant dynamism…I think with millennials in leading positions, beauty will evolve toward personalization and the concept of "made-to-measure" (a beauty for each individual) and a beauty for all types of people.

Yolanda lays out a very important point. Millennials have the power to shape the beauty industry into an even more inclusive and diverse medium as they start moving up the professional ladder. At the moment, mostly Generation Xers are leading the industry and although we are seeing an enormous positive shift in the industry, we will see a lot more in the next few years as millennials and Generation Zers move up the ranks.

Millennials are serving as a bridge between Generation X and Generation Z, whom I will talk about more in the next section. Millennials are leading today's trends since most of this generation is now in the workforce. In a few years, trends as we know them might drastically change. Generation Zers are proving to be increasingly distinct from millennials, so it will be interesting to see what they demand as they begin to have their own disposable incomes.

As suggested by Nihar Neelakanti,[80] millennials demand companies and brands that speak to them in a relevant, authentic, and genuine way. This is much different from past generations who accepted what was suggested by the beauty industry.

When speaking to the Head of Marketing LATAM at a multinational beauty company about millennials, we discussed the following:

The Zeitgeist[81] of the millennial generation is frugality. With millennials, you have a generation that is riddled with college debt, a vivid memory of the 2008 economic crash, and a desire to belong. As a result, they are discerning about what they spend their money on and the "try before you buy" feature is expected. Hence, beauty industry companies like Birchbox, Fabfitfun, Ipsy, BoxyCharm,[82] and more capitalize on the "test trial period." This enables consumers

---

80 Nihar Neelakanti is an investor at Kauffman Fellows Fund, produces The Arena Podcast, and writes the Journal Newsletter by Kauffman Fellows. Previously, he was an analyst at Correlation Ventures, which has invested in notable consumer companies such as Casper, Cotopaxi, and Imperfect Produce. He also cofounded Vendima Bags, a direct-to-consumer luxury bag startup.

81 Zeitgeist is the general mood or quality of a particular period of history, as shown by the ideas, beliefs, etc. common at the time.

82 These companies function as an online subscription service that sends its subscribers a box of a handful of selected samples of makeup or other beauty related products. The products can include skin care items, perfumes, organic based products, and various other cosmetics.

to try their products before purchasing. Millennials are more interested in trying new products, experiences, and concepts over acquiring material inventory that they might not enjoy.

The environment, political unrest, college debt, access to resources, dark aspects of technology, etc. are things that also affect the psyches of millennials and Generation Z. It is incredibly important to analyze all the distinct approaches that Generation Z, millennials, Generation X, baby boomers, and the Silent Generation, have toward life because it affects their daily consumption patterns tremendously.

Generation Z

Generation Z is the first generation to grow up with core social media platforms, Instagram and Snapchat, as these were already well-established parts of young society by the time Generation Zers got to middle school (around the ages of eleven to fourteen) and started getting smartphones. The majority of Generation Zers have grown up both with an in-person and digital personality.

This generation has grown up having digital over-stimulation and it seems that it has made them care a lot more about originality. Generation Zers are given so much information by brands, influencers, parents, friends, internet, etc. that they have made social media more about finding meaning in their own voice among the overabundance of voices they hear every day.

As Nihar Neelakanti said to me, "This has never been the case historically. Before, the ability to have a voice was reserved to a select few, but now everyone has a voice."[83] As a result, this generation wants to do anything that will give them purpose and originality and is actively looking to match with brands that will give them exactly that.

This is what prompted the "me, me, me" mentality to which niche brands have adapted well. We now see that Generation Z is beginning a new wave of trends having to do with expression and the freedom of being one's unique self. I think these trends will be beneficial to all generations because people are beginning to *feel* more represented, especially when it comes to beauty.

There remain some questions around Generation Z's purchasing behavior that will only be answered with time. Generation Z has not yet joined the workforce, so it will

---

83 Nihar Neelakanti is an investor at Kauffman Fellows Fund, produces The Arena Podcast, and writes the Journal Newsletter by Kauffman Fellows. Previously, he was an analyst at Correlation Ventures, which has invested in notable consumer companies such as Casper, Cotopaxi, and Imperfect Produce. He also cofounded Vendima Bags, a direct-to-consumer luxury bag startup.

be interesting to see whether their craving for originality will remain once they become beauty consumers on their own dime.

Will Generation Z's behavior look the same when they reach purchasing parity?

What will this originality look like?

What type of authenticity will they demand?

Generation Z and millennials are dictating the trends of today. They want to have the spotlight on themselves and on causes they care about.

As Mi Anne Chan[84] said to me, "Gen Z and millennial consumers want efficacy, and many want to consume ethically whether that means purchasing from sustainable, cruelty-free brands or from brands that have a philanthropic arm." This list of major trends of 2019 will continue to evolve in the years to come.

---

84 Mi Anne Chan is an Associate Producer and Staff Writer at Refinery29, a video director at Condé Nast entertainment, and a beauty influencer/vlogger. She has been writing, editing, filming, and making tutorials on all things beauty related since the start of her career.

CONSCIOUS OF TRENDS WE KEEP UP WITH

Inclusion & Representation

Today's consumers are powerful. They have contributed to making two non-stereotypical beauty models become some of the largest beauty influencers in the world: Huda Kattan[85] and Michelle Phan.[86] This is mainly because social media has shifted from having a defined beauty standard to owning your own identity and celebrating a more honest, authentic, and relatable beauty.

With the idea that consumers have the power to drive the beauty industry in the direction they want, there has been a wonderful switch to inclusive beauty that is seen in influencers, celebrities, models, and other key opinion leaders (KOL)s around the world. This shift has allowed the masses to see the different forms, genders, races, ethnicities, backgrounds and ages that beauty can take. As a result, beauty can now be viewed through a lens of inclusion and genuine representation, as opposed to one "standard" image of beauty. Exotic is now "in."

---

85 Huda Kattan is an Iraqi-American makeup artist, beauty blogger, and entrepreneur. She is the founder of the cosmetics line Huda Beauty and her net worth is $610 million.

86 Michelle Phan is an American makeup artist, entrepreneur, and voice actress who became notable as a YouTube personality. She is the founder of the cosmetics line EM Cosmetics, co-founder of IPSY and her net worth is $50 million.

When Talking to Nihar, we discussed brands like Haus Laboratories by Lady Gaga. This niche brand is targeting a market of people who want to *feel* beautiful and express themselves through the art of makeup. It encompasses people of any identity, gender, race, ethnicity, sexual orientation, and background.

- Haus Laboratories:[87] Lady Gaga is not just another celebrity launching her own beauty line. She is going after an under-represented market. She told *Allure*, "I want people to feel completely liberated by this line, to do whatever they want with it. Whether they wear a ton of it, buy it—or don't. I just want them to love the message. It's like just being excited that there's a party going on down the street where everybody's invited."[88] Lady Gaga and Haus laboratories believe beauty is how you see yourself.

- Fenty Beauty by Rihanna:[89] Rihanna has used her fame for a greater cause in the beauty industry. Many brands have had a hard time designing makeup for darker skin

---

87 Haus Laboratories is an inclusive, cruelty-free, and vegan cosmetic brand based on the idea of expression. It was launched by Lady Gaga in 2019.

88 "Lady Gaga And The Power Of Makeup For Allure Magazine | Tom + Lorenzo." 2019. Tom + Lorenzo. Accessed September 30, 2019. https://tomandlorenzo.com/2019/09/lady-gaga-for-allure-magazine-beauty-issue/.

89 Fenty Beauty is an inclusive cosmetic brand launched by Rihanna in 2017. Today the company is valued at $3 billion.

tones, so Fenty Beauty filled this gap in the market and made a brand targeting consumers of every skin tone or complexion.

"Natural," "Green," "Organic," and "Plant-Based"—But is it "Clean"?

People are becoming more and more aware and increasingly savvy of the ingredients they are putting on their skin, paying special attention to whether those are safe. This is changing the way consumers are buying concepts, ideas, stories, and products.

Conscious consumers now are beginning to realize that just because a product is "plant based," "natural," or "organic," does not mean the product is safe. "Clean" products, those that are safe for your skin regardless of the nature of the ingredients, are the ones that are becoming most solicited. As Paty De San Román[90] told me there is a huge change in the way we are now buying products because we care about the ethical nature of the product, we want transparency of the ingredients and formulation, and we want proof of the

---

90 Paty De San Román is the co-founder of Brand Dreamers and has been a communications and PR consultant specialized in beauty, fashion, health and lifestyle for fifteen years. She has worked on campaigns La Roche-Posay, Maria Duol, Grupo Marchon, and many others. Paty is a dreamer herself and loves communicating ideas to the greater public.

potency of a product along with knowing that it will be safe to absorb.

We love buzzwords such as "natural" and "organic."

Consumers are attracted by products that say "natural" on the label, even when there is no third third-party certification that proves its validity. Companies continue to market their brands as "natural," "clean," "green," or "organic" and continue to sell with no certifications nor evidence of these claims. These are also casting a shadow on products that are actually what they claim to be: "natural," "clean," "green," or "organic." It is completely up to us as consumers to do our homework when it comes to distinguishing the two.

For example, Clarins, the French classic luxury skin care brand that has been around since 1954, has come out with My Clarins, a new line of the brand focusing on natural ingredients. It is targeting the market that is loyal to the legitimacy and credibility of a brand like Clarins yet wants to go the more natural route.

Anti-Aging

Anti-aging is becoming a huge part of all generations from Generation Z all the way to the Silent Generation. Now, anti-aging products are not only focused on reversing the effects of aging, but also on preventing it. Anything having to do with a more youthful look is music to the consumers' ears.

Although there is a large hype on targeting the youth for these products for preventative measures, it is important that the Generation X and the Silent Generation market is being focused on, especially with the escalating life expectancy rates we have today. Only one hundred years ago, a sixty-year-old woman was considered an old person. Now, a sixty-year-old is considered middle aged and they are wanting to *feel* as beautiful as they can.

Klara Chrzuszcz[91] points out that as people continue to live longer, they will continue to care about *feeling* beautiful for longer as well. Generation X and the Silent Generation not only have the highest disposable income but are also willing to try things that will help them preserve their health and vitality. Interestingly enough, for some individuals in Generation X and the Silent Generation, the anti-aging effect of treatments is just a plus, but their main reasons for visiting professionals and getting treatments is to feel like they are getting human touch and are being taken care of.

---

91 Klara Chrzuszcz is a Medical Skin care Aesthetician, Clinical Skin care Expert, and the owner of Klara Beauty Lab. Klara is an educator in Europe for neurotoxin application as well as dermal fillers for the face and body, and she travels to teach on a yearly basis. Her approach involves delving into clients' lifestyles, diets, stress levels, etc. which, allows her to create a one-of-a-kind experience.

In one of our encounters, Klara shared a story that I will never forget. Throughout her years of working on the Upper East Side and taking care of clients from a specific demographic, she always remained honest and transparent with them as to what treatments would be beneficial to them and which were not necessary. Although her clients were able to afford visiting her on a weekly basis, she would never recommend a treatment if it was not necessary to reach the skin results they wanted.

One of Klara's clients came in to see her every other week, even after Klara had told her that she only needed to come every month. Of course, Klara was delighted to have her, but she felt the need to be truthful with the client and reiterate the fact that she didn't need to visit as often as she did. One day the client explained to Klara that her frequent visits were because being in her consultation and having her take care of her face was the most affection she received, as she felt very alone most of the time. This client's response really stuck with me and has caused me to entirely rethink a lot of why people like "beautifying themselves."

Life is short. Do what you can to live it in beauty.

The Quick Fix

The perfectly symmetrical and "dolled up" look is taking over some societies, especially among the social media generations. Surgery, fillers, and aggressive treatments that alter or enhance one's face are becoming more and more in fashion and are even becoming the norm amongst affluent people of all genders and ages. This phenomenon is especially apparent with the lip injection trend.

As Maria Eugenia Leon[92] says, "The fault comes in striving to be perfect. It is becoming normalized to modify features of your face to look like celebrities or models. This is a great danger for the younger generations, I believe. They have been introduced to a world of copious digital content, where they will have no choice but to learn to appreciate their own beauty if they want to be happy."

Clémence von Mueffling[93] adds, "Unfortunately I think people like the quick fix. We live in a society where we don't like to wait and be patient; we just want instant gratification. However, I do believe that with the right education, this can change."

---

92 Maria Eugenia Leon is the protagonist of "Blogger en Exclusiva," the Director and founder of the famous Spanish beauty blog, *Belleza en Vena*, and co-founder of *El Club de Las 11*. She writes honestly and transparently about cosmetics, perfumes, personal care, decoration, and much more.

93 Clémence von Mueffling is the Founder and Editor of Beauty and Well-Being (BWB), which brings a fresh aesthetic to the beauty and well-being media. She is also the author of *Ageless Beauty the French Way*, a luxurious, entertaining, unparalleled guide to every French beauty secret for all women.

Men's Beauty

Men's beauty is a huge untapped market that can bring many new avenues to the way men approach beauty. At one point in history, makeup and beautifying treatments were often more popular among men than women. After the eighteenth century, makeup and taking care of one's self became more associated with females. But as they say, history repeats itself. Men turn more to skin care, makeup and other beauty treatments today than they did a couple of years ago. They have begun to take care of their health and their beauty now as some become more concerned with the way they look. This trend has opened a huge new market.

We now see male-focused beauty brands telling a new story with their products. Stories all the way from those that allow men to enhance their looks while keeping their masculinity, to those that promote using makeup as a form of expression and the face as a canvas.

Pearly Whites

Hygiene and white teeth have become extremely prevalent. There is a strong correlation between healthy looking teeth/ gums and beauty. There is a large trend for having white teeth. Teeth whitening, covering your natural teeth with Veneers, and other kinds of new products are coming out to enhance our oral hygiene, health and aesthetic. Coming back to *sexual selection* that we discussed in chapter 1, oral health means youth, and youth means fertility.

Franck Moison[94] further affirms this trend saying:

> I moved twelve times since I began to work at Colgate-Palmolive and I was able to observe, interact, communicate, and commercialize products in lots of different locations. One of the most important dimensions for Colgate-Palmolive is oral health. Moving around you discover that in many cultures, oral health is directly linked to beauty. Especially because a smile is at the center of communication for many cultures. A poor smile can handicap your communication.

> The sophistication and the investment of consumers in this beauty and oral care segment is increasing with the combination of innovation and the perfect teeth trend.

> To give you an example, people today are willing to invest anywhere from five to eight hundred dollars to get their teeth whitened. In the US the teeth

---

94 Franck Moison is the former Chief Operating Officer and Vice Chairman of Colgate-Palmolive. He is an experienced Non-Executive Director with a demonstrated history of working in the consumer goods industry.

whitening segment itself is about forty percent of the oral care market, in Europe it is twenty-five percent and in Asia it is relatively high, similar to the US.

Customization and Personalization

Companies are beginning to personalize makeup and skin care, allowing people to feel like they are being cared for and that they are the curators of their beauty. These companies are giving consumers products that are catered to them, their style, their skin types, and their worries. Personalization is thriving because it is focusing on a beauty that makes an individual feel like the best version of themselves.

Moreover, consumers are looking to new technology to see faster, more potent results that are tailored to their needs. Brands must constantly think of the new formulas, gadgets, mobile apps, devices, virtual experiences, etc. that will heighten consumers' beauty experience.

Potency

Much innovation in science is happening to find the best ingredients and the most potent formulas to compete in today's saturated beauty market. A leading professional in the cosmetic fillers sphere who works for a leading global pharmaceutical company[95] noted that years ago the medical aspect of beauty was not too famous yet now it is the main and most credible aspect of the business.

Franck Moison agrees that the future of the beauty industry now relies on the science and efficacy of a product. He says companies that have science as their backbone will be around forever while others that stay relevant with their marketing or other factors cannot compare their longevity.

Colgate-Palmolive acquired EltaMD and PCA medical-grade skin care products. They made this investment because they had a commonality with their science-based business approaches. For Colgate-Palmolive, research and development is crucial. All their products are led by dentists, hygienists, or dermatologists.[96]

K Beauty

People look to South Korea for beauty innovation and formulation. This has become known as K beauty. Before, the Japanese and Europeans led the global beauty industry, but

---

95 This industry professional wishes to keep personal and company information anonymous.

96 Franck Moison is the former Chief Operating Officer and Vice Chairman of Colgate-Palmolive. He is an experienced Non-Executive Director with a demonstrated history of working in the consumer goods industry.

now South Korea has become the Silicon Valley of beauty. South Korean skin care has penetrated many different markets around the world beginning with their reputable sheet masks (Asian societies have been using sheet masks for many years), all the way to making their multi-step skin care routine the go-to for many other societies that are becoming more skin conscious.

The Natural Look

The shift to a more normal and natural look is happening. Both Dr. Alouie[97] and Dr. Barbara Sturm[98] notice a significant shift from the invasive surgical treatment space toward a more noninvasive treatment space that is also efficacious. Dr. Sturm believes there has been a recent callback to a more identity-based, natural, and unique beauty. This kind of beauty brings more confidence to women and men who are having trouble conforming to a certain beauty standard that is imposed by society.

---

97 Dr. Jouhayna Alouie is a well-known esthetician in Beirut, Paris, and Riyadh, who has been working in the field since the mid-seventies. She specializes in corrective work, permanent makeup, and enhancement facial treatments. In the past, she has worked closely with Miss France and many Arab celebrities.

98 Dr. Barbara Sturm is the founder and CEO of Dr. Barbara Sturm Molecular Cosmetics. She is a German aesthetics doctor, widely renowned for her anti-inflammatory philosophy and her non-surgical anti-aging skin treatments. Dr. Sturm translated science from her clinical research and orthopedic practice into the field of aesthetics and has been a success ever since.

WE HAVE THE POWER TO CHOOSE—
TAKE ADVANTAGE OF IT

Whether you want to get a facial enhancement or wear vegan skin care, any trend you choose to follow is your choice. Choose consciously and don't follow mindlessly.

Most trends can bring great advantages to our lives, but others are toxic for our mental health, for our physical health and for our beauty journey. One good exercise to practice is taking a step back and analyzing which trends we follow because we want to and which trends we follow because we feel like we must.

Are we aware that we are subscribing to these trends?

Are we confusing our desire to be beautiful with our desire to be accepted by society?

Even as a person who is researching, interviewing, reading books, listening to podcasts and daydreaming about the many perceptions of beauty 24/7, I need to ask myself these questions. It is easy to get carried away with the amount of information we consume on a daily basis. I find myself "brainwashed" or abiding by certain ideas or trends without analyzing them at times.

The goal of this chapter was to have you contemplate the current main trends and how different generations react to them. Because, after all, consumers are now the ones dictating the industry.

CHAPTER 4

INCLUDING ALL IN
THE CONVERSATION

———

"We are living in a time of diversity, the best possible moment to reaffirm ourselves through personal and unique beauty; without stereotypes."

—YOLANDA SACRISTÁN[99]

---

99 Yolanda Sactristán is the General Director of TheBeautyNewsroom. com and the former Editor-in-Chief of renowned publications: *Vogue* (2001-2017) and *Harper's Bazaar* (2017-2019). Yolanda is a skilled journalist with a passion for fashion, beauty, and luxury. She is always determined to produce compelling stories.

IT'S A JOURNEY

The homogenization of the standard of beauty that happened throughout the twentieth century was mostly due to the impact of Hollywood and global beauty pageants on societies all around the world. It was then further reinforced with the cultivation of beauty ideals in "the twin capitals of beauty," Paris and New York City.[100]

Now, globalization continues to press forward in yet another way. Mega brands as well as multinational corporations have now shifted and are spreading a more inclusive image of beauty.[101] The constant influx and outflux of people moving temporarily or permanently to other countries have impacted regional perceptions of beauty. As Georg von Griesheim[102] mentioned in our talk, based on the immigrational movement of populations on a global scale, all regions of the world should be preparing for a more inclusive outlook on beauty. "A huge inflow of refugees is coming into Europe, and that is changing how people perceive beauty and beautifying techniques," von Griesheim says.

---

100 "The History of Beauty." 2010. *HBS Working Knowledge.* Accessed September 30, 2019. https://hbswk.hbs.edu/item/the-history-of-beauty.

101 Ibid.

102 Georg von Griesheim is CEO of Health & Beauty, where they offer events for the manufacturing of cosmetic products, international distribution, and platforms to the professional user in a joint venture with Germany's leading people's magazine to the final consumer.

Geoffrey Jones, a Professor of Business History at the Harvard Business School, says:

> Moreover, as global firms experiment with taking new beauty ideals around the world, they are becoming agents of diffusion for different beauty ideals. L'Oréal, for example, primarily sold French brands before the 1990s. During that decade it purchased American brands such as Maybelline, Redken, and Kiehl's and globalized them. And over the last decade it has acquired Shu Uemura in Japan, Yue-Sai in China, and Britain's Body Shop. Global firms are, in this sense, now orchestrating diversity, not homogeneity.[103]

Technology, particularly digital media, has an enormous upside in this regard. It has the power to fashion a beauty image that is honest, authentic, representative, and inclusive—rather than one that starts and stays skin-deep.

I will never forget one quote that the Global Executive Director of Digital Education at a leading brand of multinational beauty company shared:[104]

---

103 "The History of Beauty." 2010. *HBS Working Knowledge.* Accessed September 30, 2019. https://hbswk.hbs.edu/item/ the-history-of-beauty.

104 This industry professional wishes to keep personal and company information anonymous.

"It's our responsibility to be an ally to the voices that are marginalized in the conversation of beauty."

This quote brought me back to my childhood. Attending so many international schools throughout my life, I had friends from Nigeria, Norway, Italy, Argentina, South Africa, the US, Spain, and Russia just to name a few. Hence, my definition of beauty was undefinable by a singular standard for the longest time. As I get older, I realize it is my duty to collaborate to the greater mission to help people see and appreciate a world with many beauties.

Accepting your local identity and expression-based beauty cultivates a positive relationship with yourself and with others. Feeling represented and part of the beauty conversation makes an enormous difference in a person's self-confidence and involvement in a community.

THE BEAUTY INDUSTRY IS ONTO SOMETHING

"When people do not feel beautiful, they lose their power."
-Bisila Bokoko[105]

---

105 Bisila Bokoko is the founder and CEO of BBES, a business development agency in New York that represents and promotes international market brands. She has inspired thousands of people and organizations around the world through conferences in which she has motivated others to pursue dreams, think big, and talk about empowerment, entrepreneurship, geopolitics, and personal branding.

If we do not *feel* beautiful, it can leave us feeling like an outcast. As Vice President of Greater China beauty business at a leading multinational corporation mentions, consumers are beginning to feel better in their own features and have more confidence in their beauty with the prominent inclusive trends that are emerging in the industry today.

VOGUE MAKES REVOLUTIONARY BREAKTHROUGH

Having lived in Mexico City for five years total, it remains one of the dearest places in my heart—especially because of its people. Mexican people, regardless of their socio-economic background, have an unexplainable beauty that has marked my life forever: the way they talk, interact with strangers, spend time with their loved ones, joke around, and their overall attitude toward life.

For this reason, when Karla Martinez de Salas[106] decided for the first time to put forth the underrepresented local beauty of Mexican society in *Vogue*, I was overjoyed. Karla Martinez de Salas spoke to me about her decision to put Yalitza

---

106 Karla Martinez de Salas is the Editor-in-Chief for *Vogue Mexico and Latin America*. She was recently included in the Business of Fashion (BoF) US list of the five hundred international fashion leaders, and since then, Karla has been in charge of the magazine's management. *Vogue Mexico and Latin America* was also awarded with best editorial content by Mexico's Fashion Digital Awards.

Aparicio Martínez,[107] on the *Vogue's* twentieth year anniversary January 2019 issue cover of *Vogue* México.

Karla said to me:

> The twentieth anniversary marks a big milestone for the magazine in Latin America. Looking at the magazines, observing and going through, I thought it was important to be more inclusive. With everything being so readily available, it's easy to look at different magazines, and all of a sudden you are stuck with the same models on every cover. I thought it was important and a good time to really do an introspection of what's happening in Mexico and Latin America and start to talk more about the things that we're doing. Representing the different types of beauty that exist in Mexico and Latin America was a focal point for sure. I think once we started talking about what we were doing and the different projects we had planned for the year, the idea to feature Yalitza Aparicio Martinez came about. This was an important moment for us because we were taking a bet on something and it ended up being the perfect step toward a more

107 Yalitza Aparicio is a Mexican actress who made her film debut as Cleo in Alfonso Cuarón's 2018 drama, *Roma*, which earned her a nomination for an Academy Award for Best Actress. *Time* magazine named her one of the one hundred most influential people in the world in 2019.

inclusive standard of beauty for *Vogue*. It was the
perfect timing with the anniversary year of *Vogue*.
It was kind of great timing as well in terms of how
to start the year.

Yalitza's cover on *Vogue's* twentieth anniversary allowed
the local Mexican population, accruing to ninety percent
according to CIA factbook, the opportunity to *feel* represented as an active participant of the beauty conversation.[108]
Yalitza appeared on the face of the December edition of
Vogue magazine wearing a Christian Dior dress next to
the title "In tiu'n ntav'i" meaning a "A star is born" in the
indigenous Mixtec language.[109]

This sends an important message to the world that underrepresented communities now have the possibility to be recognized. It is a chance to celebrate the identity-based beauty
of local Mexican skin tones, features, and pure radiance. As
Cuarón, Oscar-winning director, writes, "She focuses on
being a force of change and empowerment for indigenous

---

108 "North America: Mexico—The World Factbook—Central Intelligence
    Agency." 2019. *Cia.Gov*. Accessed October 1 2019. https://www.cia.gov/
    library/publications/the-world-factbook/geos/print_mx.html.
109 Agren, David. 2018. "'We Can Do It': Yalitza Aparicio's *Vogue*
    Cover Hailed By Indigenous Women." *The Guardian*. Accessed
    October 1 2019. https://www.theguardian.com/film/2018/dec/21/
    yalitza-aparicio-vogue-mexico-cover-roma-indigenous.

women, embracing the symbolic value of what she has done and carrying that responsibility with dignity and grace."[110]

"Other faces of Mexico are now being recognized. It is something that makes me happy and proud of my roots."

—YALITZA APARICIO

Esther Poot, an indigenous Mayan preschool teacher in the state of Quintana Roo said, "I saw it and wow! It was very powerful. Just like she did, others will say, 'We can do it. We can continue raising our voices and say yes. As indigenous women we can go on television and come out in movies or appear on the cover of a magazine.' It's exciting, but also motivating."[111]

This is the power of social approval and of societies' acceptance. We all have the right to *feel* empowered and beautiful. Yalitza, thanks to Karla Martinez de Salas' executive decision, made it possible for this to become a reality for the indigenous populations of not only Mexico, but for all of Latin America.

---

110 "Yalitza Aparicio Is On The 2019 TIME 100 List | Time.Com." 2019. *Time.Com.* Accessed August 1 2019. https://time.com/ collection/100-most-influential-people-2019/5567863/yalitza-aparicio/.

111 Agren, David. 2018. "'We Can Do It': Yalitza Aparicio's *Vogue* Cover Hailed by Indigenous Women." *The Guardian.* Accessed October 1 2019. https://www.theguardian.com/film/2018/dec/21/ yalitza-aparicio-vogue-mexico-cover-roma-indigenous.

In addition to Karla's insight, through a series of incidents, I was able to meet and speak to Yalitza herself after a talk on her struggles and her successes following the release of the film, *Roma,* at BeautyCon LA.[112]

In the Q&A section of her talk, I managed to get the attention of the man who handled the microphone standing on stage left. I felt like a kid in second grade raising my hand with the right answer to a question.

Yalitza's answer was so powerful that not only did she get emotional, but I began tearing up and soon after, every person in the audience around me. It felt like a movie.

A VOICE OF HOPE. A VOICE OF POWER. A VOICE OF BEAUTY.

My question: *What did you feel when you saw yourself for the first time on the front cover of Vogue? What did it make you feel about your beauty and about the beauty of indigenous women in Mexico?*

Yalitza Aparicio responded to my question with the following:

---

112 *Roma,* the film, is a semi-autobiographical take on Cuarón's upbringing, set in 1970-71 in the Colonia Roma neighborhood of Mexico City, stars Yalitza Aparicio and Marina de Tavira and follows the life of a live-in housekeeper of a middle-class family in Mexico.

It made me quite nervous to be on the cover of the December 2018 issue of *Vogue*. When I received this invitation, I simply told them, "Yes, yes, yes!" as I answered to everything that was happening to me at that time. For me, it was all so surreal that I didn't realize it was actually happening to me. When we arrived at the photo session and I saw everything set up for the shoot, I understood, "Oh yes, this really is happening."

When I held the magazine in my hands for the first time, it made me very excited...(starts stuttering and her voice begins to crack)...because for the first time ...(stops talking for five seconds from overwhelming emotion and all the crowd begins to cheer).

For the first time, people who had grown up with the same idea I had of life and beauty standards were seeing a representation of themselves on the cover of a top beauty and fashion magazine. And not only in any magazine's cover, but *Vogue's*. And when I saw the comments, that was what I liked the most, they thanked me for representing them on a cover.

An overwhelming amount of people still feel ostracized from the conversation of beauty today and it is our duty as citizens of the world to include them. Inclusion in beauty is not a "should" but a "must."

Speaking to the woman who made this step forward in the representation of indigenous people in beauty was very moving.

In the video that *Vogue* shot for her, *Yalitza Aparicio en la Portada de Vogue México—Enero 2019.* She says:

> As a strong woman, I have been able to be an inspiration for other people. Nowadays stereotypes are being broken that only certain people can aspire to be on the cover of a magazine like *Vogue*, an icon of beauty, or an actress. Other faces of Mexico are now being recognized and it makes me very happy and proud of my roots. They help me to feel beautiful without forgetting my origin. You have to keep fighting to get what you want in life.[113]

Giving indigenous people representation in the beauty industry is not only a step forward in allowing all women to *feel* beautiful, but also a political advancement. It is fostering more confidence for people to reach their maximum potential and to push society be the best it can be.

---

113 "Yalitza Aparicio En La Portada De *Vogue* México—Enero 2019." 2019. *YouTube.* Accessed October 1 2019. https://www.youtube. com/watch?v=SmEhcDZqrUo.

"Beauty is not skin deep. It goes far beyond that," as Klara Chrzuszcz[114] stated in our talk. What your presence makes people around you feel and the energy you transcend to others matters.

Valentina Collado Rojas[115] outlined the strides taken to push *Vogue* toward a more inclusive space for its twentieth anniversary, "We are living in times when all types of beauties must be celebrated. Our current societies are demanding for models to come in unique, authentic, and real forms, so much so that Yalitza Aparicio's *Vogue* cover had the highest demand of any other magazine in Mexico."

Yalitza's face has given light to the conversation of indigenous beauty in Latin America, where there is an enormous consumer market that falls under this category. Both for justice and profit purposes, leaving indigenous people out of the local perception of beauty is a definite loss for all.

---

114 Klara Chrzuszcz is a Medical Skin care Aesthetician, Clinical Skin care Expert, and the owner of Klara Beauty Lab. Klara is an educator in Europe for neurotoxin application as well as dermal fillers for the face and body, and she travels to teach on a yearly basis. Her approach involves delving into clients' lifestyles, diets, stress levels, etc. which, allows her to create a one-of-a-kind experience.

115 Valentina Collado Rojas is the Fashion Editor and Stylist of *Vogue Mexico & Latin America*. She was previously an Assistant for Special Events Department at Vogue Condé Nast Americas. She is experienced in Editorial and Fashion Styling, Event Planning, Online/New Media, PR, and Sales industries.

PUBLIC REACTION

When asked about the public's reaction, Karla Martinez de Salas stated:

I think the public's reaction was incredibly positive. It was an absolute hit. A much more positive feedback than we ever imagined it would be. At the beginning, there was significant criticism. But in general, all the reactions were really, really, really positive all over the world.

It is surreal, and we can't believe it finally was able to happen. It is something we are very proud and happy about.

When I first arrived at *Vogue*, I was told something along the lines of: we shoot models here—high profile models. That's what people expect from us. But now, we have done people like Camilla Cabello, Litza Veloz, and Yalitza Aparicio. People are tired of seeing the same things everywhere and want to feel represented. I feel like people were really excited when we started doing more local images of beauty. They felt more in tune with what we were putting out.

In May 2019, for example, we had Christy Turlington and Marina de Tavira, Mexican actresses both over the age of forty. They look amazing, but they're not heavily retouched. In April, we have a plus size model. I think we are just being more representative in general. We are reaching for a more inclusive representation of beauty.

Valentina said, "We are now in a very important moment where ethnic factions are now being accepted in the high fashion world." She explained that in all the Fashion Weeks she had attended in previous years she had seen a tremendous shift in the choice of models on the runway. She says now there are stunning women from all colors, all features, and all ethnicities walking Fashion Week, something that was not prominent until recently.

"I think *Vogue*, for a lot of people, is a style, beauty and cultural reference. So, I think it's important we show a break from former stereotypes of beauty and make sure to provide what people want to see."

—KARLA MARTINEZ DE SALAS

Latina local beauty, in this case, is beginning to be put forward on many magazine covers now that *Vogue* has broken the seal. This initiative of inclusive beauty has been made in the beauty industry, but it is only the beginning.

THE 360° VIEW OF BEAUTY

Meeting people with different ethnicities, cultures, and perspectives allows us to see the world through a new set of lenses. Inclusivity is all about learning about other cultures; not just seeing a cocktail of different skin tones on billboards, but actually getting to know people, understanding where they come from and where they want to go.

Social media and technology have afforded us a 360 panoramic view of what other beauties are out there without having to spend a dime on travel. Social media has pushed for a more inclusive understanding of beauty amongst all smartphone owners. Seeing all the different faces, features, skin tones, and forms that beauty can embody also helps us get out of the habit of seeing beauty as something tangible. *So many faces of beauty are out there, so how could there ever be anything like a concrete standard of beauty?*

As little as twenty years ago, no one would have ever imagined that an estimated 2.7 billion people in the world would have access to a smartphone and instantly be exposed to content that could broaden perspectives in a way that no other medium has ever been able to do.[116] It is mind-blowing

---

116 "Number of Smartphone Users Worldwide 2014–2020 | Statista." 2019. *Statista*. Accessed October 1 2019. https://www.statista.com/statistics/330695/number-of-smartphone-users-worldwide/.

that we have the luxury today to open our phones, and in a split second we have all sorts of beauty out there.

As the *NYT* mentions in "Beauty Is More Diverse Than Ever. But Is It Diverse Enough?" "Younger, older, darker, lighter, different undertones—you should be able to look at the face in front of you and match." This is one of the main reasons why pop star Rihanna's Fenty line had such success with her brand that is well-known for launching the forty-foundations standard, giving the industry a new standard to follow.[117]

In this way companies can see where underrepresentation is happening in order to represent and fill that market—a win-win. It is an unquestionable fact that all skin tones, complexions, ethnicities, ages, genders, and identities need to be represented in beauty brands if they want to resonate with the consumers of today.[118]

DIVERSITY AND INCLUSION

Diversity and inclusion are becoming **musts** in almost all industries. Genuine and intentional inclusivity in the workforce is necessary for all companies to thrive. If no one

---

117 "Beauty Is More Diverse Than Ever. But Is It Diverse Enough?" 2019. Nytimes.Com. Accessed October 1 2019. https://www. nytimes.com/2018/09/11/style/beauty-diversity.html.

118 Ibid.

behind the scenes looks like the consumers who are buying products, how can we expect to get products catered to them?

Consumers *feel* comfortable with a beauty brand when the employees of the brand are just as diverse as who they are selling to. Kennedy Daniel[119] is a big proponent of this theory too. Kennedy points out that Glossier was so successful in attracting women from all backgrounds because the work environment behind the scenes was just as inclusive and uplifting as their products and mission.

While speaking with Jordana Shiau,[120] she agreed with this as well. She, however, discussed with me the other side— the misfortune that the beauty industry is still very whitewashed. Especially in corporate, it is still predominantly white male-dominated. But you do see it changing.

Jordana says:

> I've worked on the corporate side of large beauty companies before, where you have the people who

---

119 Kennedy Daniel works part time at Glossier LA on Melrose Place as an Offline Editor while she finishes her BA at the University of Southern California. Kennedy is proud to say she was a member of the original team of Offline Editors who helped open the store in the Spring of 2018.

120 Jordana Shiau is a Manager of Social and Digital Strategy at Laura Mercier. She has been in the corporate side of the beauty industry for the last five years working from startups to the largest beauty brands in the world.

are super corporate and have been there for years. These people usually wear pencil skirts, heels, a tie, and are usually middle-aged white women and men. But then, you have the younger generation of adults coming into the beauty industry, moving into the more digital, social, and PR roles. That's a whole other demographic of diversity.

It's kind of weird because you have these old school people who have been here for years and like to do things a certain way and stick to traditional media, and then you have a bunch of kids coming in like me with crazy orange hair, with all different skin tones and a more relatable sense to inclusive beauty of today.

We are now having to explain that not everything is so cookie cutter anymore and there's so many new ways to reach your consumer in a more relevant way than a TV commercial or a print ad. Quite honestly it is a cool time to be in the industry because two very different groups are working behind beauty companies at the moment. The younger generations are really pushing for inclusivity and succeeding at it.

There is a lot of disingenuous diversity and inclusion at the moment to "fill quotas." In my opinion this is not helping the long-term conversation of inclusivity, productivity, and efficacy in the workforce. As Sam Fine, a makeup artist known for working with Naomi Campbell, Iman, and Queen Latifah, says, "We're stuck in a place that is 'politically correct.'"[121]

"Beauty Is More Diverse Than Ever. But Is It Diverse Enough?" could not have stated this any better:

> For example, every brand is launching forty foundation colors now because it's the trendy thing to do. But is the brand actually doing the work—the initiatives and outreach? The stock needs to be there, and not only forty shades at your Times Square store. The people at the counter need training.[122]

"Diversity is being invited to the party; inclusion is being asked to dance."[123]

—BOZOMA SAINT JOHN[124]

---

121 "Beauty Is More Diverse Than Ever. But Is It Diverse Enough?." 2019. Nytimes.Com. Accessed October 1 2019. https://www.nytimes.com/2018/09/11/style/beauty-diversity.html.

122 Ibid.

123 Ibid.

124 Bozoma Saint John is an American businesswoman and Chief Marketing Officer at William Morris Endeavor.

One of the reasons for the enormous success of Fenty by Rihanna was due to its genuine inclusivity in all aspects of the brand marketing, product, stock, models, employees, outreach, and DNA of the brand.

Ariane Hunter[125] said to me:

> Fenty Beauty, Rihanna's line, is a great example of an inclusive beauty. Not only is her makeup line brilliant and inclusive of all shades and all beauties, but her social media campaign was really well done in terms of the pictures and the models she chose to represent the line. I think it was very much in alignment with the brand or the message she wanted to convey.
>
> It's comforting when you see a model who even slightly looks like you because it almost gives you permission to be yourself and feel beautiful.
>
> I think technology has helped a lot in the democratization of the perception of beauty. Like with everything, though, there are drawbacks as well. I

---

125 Ariane Hunter is the CEO and founder of Project She Went For Her Dreams—a personal branding and marketing firm in New York City, serving clients globally. She works with enlightened women and businesses to develop creative brands and build artistic marketing strategies to stand out in a meaningful, authentic way.

don't think there's anything wrong with enhancing your beauty and making visible what you already have, but there is a fine line that needs to be clear between that and tampering with your own inner and outer beauty. Always make sure the energy and the intention behind it is not to fill a void or wanting to fit in, rather than to feel like a better version of yourself. Bring mindfulness to the way you treat your beauty.

As Mi Anne Chan[126] mentions, "Social media is giving consumers a microphone to tell brands exactly what they want from their products. It's allowing consumers to call out brands for neglecting shade ranges or ask brands why their packaging isn't sustainable. It's given consumers the opportunity to tell brands who they want to see represented." For there to be true inclusion in beauty companies, there needs to be more communication with the consumer.

Diversity and Inclusion executed with intention will allow the industry to progress in a direction that is created BY all beauties FOR all beauties.

---

126 Mi Anne Chan is an Associate Producer and Staff Writer at Refinery29, a video director at Condé Nast entertainment, and a beauty influencer/vlogger. She has been writing, editing, filming, and making tutorials on all things beauty related since the start of her career.

BRIDGING THE GAP

Sephora launched a new platform called "We Belong to Something Beautiful" in May 2019 with the mission of creating marketing for beauty that is more genuinely inclusive.[127]

The platform's motto is: "Sephora believes in championing all beauty, living with courage, and standing fearlessly together to celebrate our differences. We will never stop building a community where diversity is expected, self-expression is honored, all are welcome, and you are included." [128]

As Sephora shows to be doing, the beauty industry can act as a bridge to connect societies. Bisila Bokoko[129] mentions:

> Beauty has become a political statement, making ingredients and societies more inclusive. Populism in political areas is separating people and now beauty is

---

127 "Here's the Important Reason Sephora Is Closing All Its Stores For An Hour On June 5." 2019. *Bustle*. Accessed October 1 2019. https://www.bustle.com/p/sephoras-we-belong-to-something-beautiful-pledge-further-proves-the-brands-commitment-to-diversity-17911715.

128 Stuart, Eden. 2019. "Sephora Commits To Inclusivity With Platform, Manifesto." *Global Cosmetic Industry*. Accessed October 1 2019. https://www.gcimagazine.com/marketstrends/channels/other/Sephora-Commits-to-Inclusivity-with-Platform-Manifesto-510510391.html.

129 Bisila Bokoko is the founder and CEO of BBES, a business development agency in New York that represents and promotes international market brands. She has inspired thousands of people and organizations around the world through conferences in which she has motivated others to pursue dreams, think big, and talk about empowerment, entrepreneurship, geopolitics, and personal branding.

bringing people together and making people feel more unified. Beauty is a tool to make the world a more inclusive place. Women do not have to look a certain way to get married and have a family. Now passion and brains are more beautiful than any other look.

Feeling beautiful bridges us all together, and it makes us human—sometimes even what pushes individuals to hold onto a part of themselves during hard times.

"DON'T HATE ME BECAUSE I'M BEAUTIFUL"

Not only racial groups but other previously marginalized groups such as the LGBTQIA+ community are equally important for the beauty industry to include. The industry has made considerable strides in the last couple of years to make sure and include them in the conversation too.

A great example of this is P&G's Pantene, previously known for ensuring "beautiful hair" with their products. Pantene made it a mission not only to include all genders, races, ethnicities, and identities, but specifically the LGBTQ+ community as well with their "Don't Hate Me Because I'm Beautiful LGBTQ+ ad" campaign.[130]

130 Size, Full, Full Size, Full Size, and BUSINESS WIRE. 2019. "Pantene Launches "Don't Hate Me Because I'M #Beautifulgbtq" To Redefine What 'Beautiful' Looks Like Today." *Businesswire. Com.* Accessed October 1 2019. https://www.businesswire.com/news/home/20190618005209/en/.

Ilaira Resta, Vice President, North America Hair Care, Procter & Gamble said that 60 percent of LGBTQ+ persons change their hair when they have a life or identity change. It is a significant component of their "transformation moment." For this reason, "Pantene wants every head of hair held high with pride and encourages the LGBTQ+ community and its allies to express their authentic selves and share their own transformations to show the world all they are capable of and just what "beautiful" looks like."[131]

This campaign was comprised of a video of beautiful LGBTQIA+ community members modeling, dancing, and radiating the most incredible energy with their fabulous hair. This line of meaningful work highlights a brand value system that can ensure longevity and loyalty from consumers. Pantene was one of the pioneers that put a focus on authentic inclusion of the LGBTQIA+ community.

BOYS, BOYS, BOYS

The stigma that it is not masculine for men to care about their skin and general appearance is about to be over. Now, it is encouraged to open up the market to the other major gender of the world's population. Estimates say the men's personal care industry will hit $166 billion by 2022, according to Allied

---

131 Ibid.

Market Research.[132] Just last year, men's skin care products alone saw more than a seven percent jump in sales and the category and is currently valued at $122 million, according to market researcher NPD Group.[133]

The market for male skin care is a multibillion-dollar growth opportunity. I believe it will turn the stigma of men's grooming into a more normalized and even necessary—just like shaving! Not only will they be shaving and doing all the other things they already do, but also taking care of their skin.

For men, taking care of their skin is important to ensure they treat their necessities like irritation from shaving and protecting their skin from sun damage and pollution. In addition, many products that have been previously marketed to women such as serums, face oils, toners, and creams will also be targeted for men. I believe this will make them feel like they belong in this domain.

---

132 Warfield, Nia. 2019. "Men Are A Multibillion Dollar Growth Opportunity For The Beauty Industry." *CNBC*. Accessed October 1 2019. https://www.cnbc.com/2019/05/17/men-are-a-multibillion-dollar-growth-opportunity-for-the-beauty-industry.html.

133 Ibid.

Dr. Barbara Sturm,[134] for example, has a well-established men's skin care line that is straightforward, simple, and effective. Although the industry is pushing into the male beauty market, a lot of male consumers are still predominantly from the LGBTQIA+ community. Straight men are having a harder time transitioning into it, but they will.

Men are less likely to be steered toward skin care because often they don't think taking care of skin is for men. They don't know the correct products to use or how to use them, and they are frequently shy about asking women or even looking it up themselves in fear of losing masculinity.

Then incredible male makeup artists are now expressing themselves and their identity through makeup. These men are making makeup a lot more gender fluid and changing some preconceptions we previously had on the functions of makeup. Byrdie says, "Male beauty influencers like Coverboy James Charles and beauty mogul Jeffree Star have shown that makeup is in the early stages of becoming more gender-inclusive. This concept, however, is hardly new."

---

134 Dr. Barbara Sturm is the founder and CEO of Dr. Barbara Sturm Molecular Cosmetics. She is a German aesthetics doctor, widely renowned for her anti-inflammatory philosophy and her non-surgical anti-aging skin treatments. Dr. Sturm translated science from her clinical research and orthopedic practice into the field of aesthetics and has been a success ever since.

Maybe it is new, but only for the generations of today. As mentioned in chapter 1, before the makeup industry became a female-exclusive business after the eighteenth century, men actually used makeup as well.[135] The church then long considered makeup "an abomination" creating a diffused idea around it of vanity, femininity, and "the Devil's work."[136] Therefore the masculine approach to makeup was lost.

Now it is all fair game, and this male beauty market is coming in HOT!

GETTING MEN'S ATTENTION

Peter Thomas Roth[137] made a question that seemed complex a lot simpler: "How do I attract all genders to my products?" Peter says, "Just make it gender neutral."

---

135 "From 4000 BCE To Today: The Fascinating History of Men And Makeup." 2019. *Byrdie.* Accessed October 1 2019. https://www.byrdie.com/history-makeup-gender#targetText=For percent20millenniapercent2C percent

136 "The History of Male Makeup." 2012. *Infashuationdotnet. Wordpress.Com.* Accessed October 1 2019. https://infashuationdotnet.wordpress.com/2012/12/07/mens-makeup/.

137 Peter Thomas Roth is the CEO, founder, and formulator of Peter Thomas Roth Clinical Skin Care, is an influential segment leader in the beauty industry and continues to corner the clinical market as a groundbreaking, results-focused innovator. Today, Peter's comprehensive range of products are sold worldwide in over eighty countries, with Peter leading all research and development efforts at his state-of-the-art lab and manufacturing facility.

Peter says all his products are gender neutral except for a few mascaras that are targeted toward women. When he formulates and manufactures products, he wouldn't put anything on the market that he wouldn't use himself.

Although it is relevant for your specific target market to feel represented by a brand's message and packaging, it is important to realize that the potency and the formulation of products for men and women are mostly the same. The largest difference is the way they are packaged—lighter colors for females and darker ones for males.

Peter prefers fragrance-free products or slightly fragranced products if need be, which thereby make them gender neutral. He believes once you start layering heavily fragranced serums and creams, the scents will compete. Peter feels the fragrance you and people around you smell should be the fragrance or cologne you choose, not that of your skin care.

If you have been in the predicament before, doubting whether to use a product that does not look like it is catered for your gender, try to detach from that idea. Especially with skin care; if it is quality, it should be just as potent and effective on your skin no matter your gender. Good skin care masterminds know skin, and skin knows no gender.

The general sentiment is that men and women shop the same. Well, they don't!

Peter also mentions that women tend to frequent the store more often than men, so they see the newest products and fashion and pick these out for men. At the same time, the male beauty market can be a multilayered one because although it is being marketed for men, many women still shop for them. Thus the marketing and packaging must attract a woman in order for them to want to buy it for men.

For this reason, Peter says that when it comes to the male consumer, there are two main types of male skin care consumers. Some will have their significant other buy products for them, and others have skin issues and are genuinely interested in solving them. The latter tend to do their research well, getting information from doctors, friends, beauty advisors, magazines, blogs, etc. to find what works best. Many men, however, aren't as concerned with their skin care needs and just tend to use whatever products are available, be it shampoo to wash their face or their significant other's moisturizer.

The beauty industry has now found a huge window of opportunity with the male market that will keep strengthening over the next few years.

WHY SO ANTI-AGING?

I am a proponent of aging gracefully, but it takes a lot of dedication. If you want to remain beautiful all your life, you shouldn't be scared of aging but rather of losing your inner radiance.

"Beauty is about making someone feel and look like the best version of themselves at all stages of their life."

—CLÉMENCE VON MUEFFLING[138]

Elder women can show signs of age yet still radiate an unexplainable energy, like my grandmother Teresa did. My beautiful grandmother radiated an energy that would make all people smile when they looked at her, and on top of this, she took care of her skin, nails, hair, eyebrows, and more. She was a true beauty queen. Aging gracefully means aging with humor and not taking yourself too seriously and is part of eternal beauty.

I believe it is imperative to value aging in the conversation of beauty, especially when speaking about women. In the world of women, we have been brainwashed to categorize age into beautiful twenties, motherhood thirties, aging forties and

---

138 Clémence von Mueffling is the Founder and Editor of Beauty and Well-Being (BWB), which brings a fresh aesthetic to the beauty and well-being media. She is also the author of *Ageless Beauty the French Way*, a luxurious, entertaining, unparalleled guide to every French beauty secret for all women.

fifties, old sixties and so on. Unlike other stigmas discussed earlier that are successfully becoming more included in the beauty conversation, age is not doing so well.

Our image of beauty is geared toward youth, which brings us back to the sexual selection from chapter 1. But the real reason for us to be attracted toward youth is not exactly just because of age. It is more due to the healthy radiance one transmits when they are young, which usually means they are fertile. For this reason, if we maintain the health of our body and mind and work to take care of our bodies, no age can beat our emanating beauty.

It is our duty to understand the beauty that lies in the elder generations. This beauty is not the same as when we are in our twenties. Elder beauty comes from health, happiness and profound life experience.

In 2016, Lancôme, brought timeless beauty back with Isabella Rossellini at age sixty-three. She is an Italian actress, director and style icon, who was the first face of the beauty house "Lancôme woman" in 1983. Isabella Rossellini, fourteen years after becoming the face of Lancôme was asked to step down since she was not as young as they would have liked her to be. Recently, she was taken back in hopes of helping the modern age-inclusive perception of beauty. *Fashion Network* says, "She also maintains a very positive, serene attitude to age, which she experiences as liberating and self-affirming."[139]

Isabella Rossellini says, "I am well aware that this decision goes well beyond me. It's a strong indication of Lancôme's inclusiveness and celebration of all women."[140]

We should talk about "anti-aging" in a more positive light instead of seeing it as "not becoming old." I personally don't like that term. I think a healthier way to approach the world of anti-aging is to refer to it as the maintenance of glow, radiance, or grace.

Anti-aging has such a negative connotation because it means we believe aging is undesirable. This very belief steers some people in the direction of exaggerated cosmetic treatments and surgeries. As Klara Chrzuszcz[141] says, "We have incredible options to help clients age

---

139 "Isabella Rossellini Returns to Lancôme." 2016. *Fashionnetwork. Com.* Accessed October 1 2019. https://ww.fashionnetwork.com/news/Isabella-Rossellini-returns-to-Lancome,665917.html#. XXPTui2B124.

140 Ibid.

141 Klara Chrzuszcz is a Medical Skin care Aesthetician, Clinical Skin care Expert, and the owner of Klara Beauty Lab. Klara is an educator in Europe for neurotoxin application as well as dermal fillers for the face and body, and she travels to teach on a yearly basis. Her approach involves delving into clients' lifestyles, diets, stress levels, etc. which, allows her to create a one-of-a-kind experience.

gracefully. I do believe maintenance is key and creating a regimen that works with your lifestyle is important to age with radiance!"

You might be thinking: Well yes, but, there is really no such thing as "aging gracefully." Sagging is not too graceful. Especially for women, at fifty, you are having hot flashes, you are tired, you have mood swings, your lashes are thin, your skin is lifeless, and you have huge bags under your eyes, etc. This is not wrong, but it is easy to list all the physical changes one sees. The thing to understand is that it's not about the signs of aging. It's about how you handle them and how you present yourself and your beauty.

Always remember that you are a compilation of your experiences, wisdom, and your inner beauty as you age. That is true beauty. I hope this definition of true beauty will be more promoted in the beauty industry in the years to come. We are all living longer, and we are going to be older for the better part of our existence. We are doing ourselves a disservice by thinking youth is equal beauty; it is simply a different beauty.

Think of healthy aging as beauty.

TOP INCLUSIVE BRANDS IN ALL REGIONS

All statistics below are in terms of Earned Media Value, or EMV, which is Tribe Dynamics'[142] proprietary metric for quantifying the estimated value of consumer engagement with digital earned media.

Rising Gender-Neutral Brands (according to CEW)[143]

1. Non-Gender Specific "NGS" (Clean Gender-Neutral Skincare)
2. Fluide (Makeup for Everyone)
3. Context Gender Neutral Skincare)
4. Jecca Blac (Gender Neutral Contouring and Concealers)
5. Panacea Skincare (High-Quality Gender-Neutral Skincare)
6. Asarai (Naturopath-developed Gender-Neutral Skincare)

---

142 Tribe Dynamics' proprietary data and digital expertise focus on measurement of social influence within the beauty, fashion, and lifestyle industries.

143 "Rising Gender-Neutral Brands—Cosmetic Executive Women." 2019. Cosmetic Executive Women. Accessed October 8 2019. https://www.cew.org/beauty_news/rising-gender-neutral-brands/.

Top Beauty Brands Q2 2019 (Tribe Dynamics)[144]

US

1. Anastasia Beverly Hills
2. Huda Beauty
3. ColourPop Cosmetics
4. Benefit
5. Morphe
6. MAC
7. Fenty Beauty
8. Too Faced
9. NYX Professional Makeup
10. Tarte

Korea

1. YSL (Beauty)
2. Dior (Beauty)
3. Innisfree
4. Chanel (Beauty)
5. Clio
6. MAC
7. Etude House
8. 3CE
9. Bobbi Brown
10. Benefit

---

144 "Tribe Dynamics: Top Indie Brands Of Q2 2019—Cosmetic Executive Women." 2019. *Cosmetic Executive Women.* Accessed November 3 2019. https://www.cew.org/beauty_news/tribe-dynamics-indie-beauty-debrief-for-q2-2019/.

Japan

1. Dior
2. CANMAKE Tokyo
3. Chanel (Beauty)
4. YSL (Beauty)
5. Shiseido
6. MAC
7. Kate Tokyo
8. L'Oréal Paris
9. NARS
10. Opera

France

1. Too Faced
2. NYX Professional Makeup
3. L'Oréal Paris
4. YSL (Beauty)
5. MAC
6. Huda Beauty
7. Anastasia Beverly Hills
8. Dior (Beauty)
9. Fenty Beauty
10. Benefit

UK

1. Huda Beauty
2. Anastasia Beverly Hills
3. MAC
4. Benefit
5. NYX Professional Makeup
6. NARS
7. Fenty Beauty
8. Morphe
9. Too Faced
10. Revolution Beauty

Australia

1. Benefit
2. MAC
3. Anastasia Beverly Hills
4. Huda Beauty
5. Too Faced
6. Fenty Beauty
7. Tarte
8. NARS
9. Hourglass
10. ColourPop

Gulf Countries

1. Benefit
2. MAC
3. Huda Beauty
4. Makeup Forever
5. Fenty Beauty
6. Dior (Beauty)
7. NARS
8. Too Faced
9. Anastasia Beverly Hills
10. NYX Professional Makeup

TOP Skincare Brands: Tribe Dynamics shared the top skin care brands for May 2019[145]

1. Tatcha
2. Farsáli (Skincare)
3. Pixi Beauty (Skincare)
4. Ole Henriksen
5. Kylie Skin
6. Fresh
7. Glamglow
8. Drunk Elephant
9. Glow Recipe
10. L'Oréal Paris

---

145 "Tribe Dynamics: August's Top 10 Cosmetics, Skin Care And Hair Brands On Social—Cosmetic Executive Women." 2019. *Cosmetic Executive Women*. Accessed November 3 2019. https://www.cew.org/beauty_news/tribe-dynamics-augusts-top-10-cosmetics-skin-care-and-hair-brands-on-social/.

CHAPTER 5

CONNECTING WITH YOURSELF AND THE RIGHT INGREDIENTS

FEELING BEAUTIFUL IS DIRECTLY RELATED TO YOUR HEALTH

Growing up with Basque parents, food was a sacred part of life—nutritious foods of course. One of the greatest excitements of going to see my grandparents every summer or winter break was to have my grandmothers cook the most incredible Spanish meals. Nowadays, I have this same exact feeling about going home to my own mother's food. I cannot help but think of the aroma when I enter my parents' home of fresh home-cooked Mediterranean meals. Even my friends recognize this smell. My mom has always been an incredible chef and both my parents are and have always been cautious about what my sister and I put in our bodies, stressing the Mediterranean diet and teaching us about the importance of healthy and nutritious foods. They believe this is the only true way to a successful lifestyle.

Only much later was I finally able to internalize the significance of what they had been telling me since I was a little girl. Eating the right things makes it a lot easier to cultivate that inner beauty.

In my junior year of high school, I went through a rough spell with a sphincter[146] malfunction. This contraption makes sure food goes from the esophagus to your stomach. After many doctor visits, I realized I had a severe case of GERD (Gastroesophageal Reflux Disease) and a Hiatal hernia to add the cherry on top. I was swallowing about six pills of medication every day to subside the effects of these complications and help my body do what it was supposed to naturally do.

After a lot of analysis and being warned that this case of GERD could potentially cause esophageal or throat cancer in years to come, my family and I decided it was best to

---

146 A sphincter is a circular muscle that maintains constriction and relaxes around a body passage or orifice as required by normal physiological functioning.

go through a fundoplication surgery for GERD. This meant I could stop living on my daily dose of pills to treat my incessant reflux and grant me a more enjoyable normal life. During this time, I hurt so much every time I ate I had to be hyper aware of what I ingested. I was not well.

What I didn't know was that this would be a turning point in my life. Having the surgery was the best decision my parents and I could have made. Besides the tough surgery and some long-term side effects that I can live with, it had miraculously freed me of the constant discomfort that distracted me from living my life as I wanted. I was finally able to focus on myself, my well-being, and my inner beauty.

After this, I became more aware of the signals my body gave me. I researched endlessly about different foods, ingredients, and workouts that fit my lifestyle. Ultimately, this served me to learn what was right for me.

Not only has this shift in my life allowed me to *feel* more beautiful inside, but also it has visibly improved my skin, making it healthier and more radiant. People tell me all the time that my skin is glowing and always ask me what I do to my skin. Honestly, it is not one thing I do. It is my holistic approach to beauty. It is a work in progress, and I try my best to make the best decisions for myself every day without being extreme or obsessive.

HOLISTIC APPROACH

Mindfulness, skin care, sleep, meditation, clean ingredients, detox, and silent retreats are all examples of how our society is becoming more interested in getting our body, mind, and soul to be at ease and working as one. All these examples Paty De San Roman[147] and I discussed while we spoke about indirect avenues to a more holistic form of beauty. All these trends are really trying to make us feel good from the root.

Yalda Alaoui[148] could not have said it better:

> Beauty reflects health, which is linked to how well both our body and mind are. Health is an all-encompassing concept and I firmly believe beauty comes from within. It isn't about "perfection" but about how radiant and healthy you look and how happy and positive you are with yourself. The most beautiful people to me, are not the ones who have a "perfect plastic" but those who radiate this energy I am referring to.

147 Paty De San Román is the co-founder of Brand Dreamers and has been a communications and PR consultant specialized in beauty, fashion, health and lifestyle for fifteen years. She has worked on campaigns La Roche-Posay, Maria Duol, Grupo Marchon, and many others. Paty is a dreamer herself and loves communicating ideas to the greater public.

148 Yalda Alaoui is the Founder of Eat Burn Sleep. Yalda was diagnosed in 2007 with two auto-immune diseases—Ulcerative Colitis and Auto-Immune Haemolytic Anaemia—that made her begin to extensively research nutrition and health. A ten-year period of research and recovery led her to share her knowledge and make a full career change in order to help more people.

Since I have gotten my health back after overcoming two serious auto-immune conditions, Ulcerative Colitis and Auto-Immune Hemolytic Anaemia, whenever I stick to the Eat Burn Sleep lifestyle I have created, which includes having fun and being social, people now comment on how well and healthy I look! It is a great reminder for me to keep on track and to look after my body, my mind and my friends!

Yalda is proof that a holistic approach to beauty can be the most satisfying of all. She not only talked about her food lifestyle being a key component of her health and well-being, but also taking care of physical health and her mental health by keeping her relationships alive and well because this is what allows beauty to shine.

As Dr. Sturm says:

Everyone has some idea of the perfect way to a healthy lifestyle and a holistic form of beauty—eat healthy, don't drink, don't smoke—but for some reason everyone is messing up the skin, throwing all these super harsh ingredients on it. They don't keep in mind that everything they put on their skin goes into their entire system. I do my best to educate and inform people about all these things.

Understanding the principle behind the mind and body connection often determines our well-being and how we look and *feel* about ourselves. In many ways, our skin reflects our state of mind. "When our mind and body are in sync, this harmonious state of balance has a profound effect on our appearance, allowing radiance and confidence to come forth," as Ewelina Aiossa[149] expressed to me.

Inner turmoils such as stress, lack of sleep, anxiousness, sadness, etc. always reveal themselves on the surface of our skin in the form of skin complications, fine lines, skin dullness, and more while inner-peace and a positive mindset bring forth a brighter complexion and relaxed facial expressions. Ewelina also points out that beauty goes from the outside in. Seventy percent of everything you apply on your skin gets absorbed to some degree into your body and often travels to your bloodstream or lymphatic system. If the substance happens to be toxic, it can cause alterations to your hormones, which can alter the way we perceive and feel.

Looking good often depends on feeling good. Therefore, it is important to be mindful of what we apply to our skin. We need to think: Is this product benefiting a state of health or

---

149 Ewelina Aiossa is the Assistant Vice President of Marketing at SkinCeuticals, L'Oreal. She serves on UBM—Dermatology Times Industry Council and SkinCeuticals (SC) Leadership Team panel. She has a strong knowledge of the aesthetic business, professional channel, products, and ingredients.

disturbing the balance? The cleaner, safer and free of nasties the product is, the better.

Another example Ewelina gave me is the use of essential oils. In the pursuit of beauty and wellness, more people are embracing self-care and incorporating mood-enhancing products that integrate essential oils. This illustrates how important it is for everything to work in unison. You should look at beauty as more than just products you put on your face, but how these products make you feel. Your skin is the largest organ of your body, and when you internalize this fact, you start being more aware of how you treat it.

A well-known nutritionist and holistic beauty practitioner in Los Angeles,[150] mentioned the importance of exercise for our complexion and mindset:

> It is a misconception that working out or moving our bodies is a "healthy lifestyle." It is something we should all be doing as a "normal" part of our everyday live the same way we need nutrition every day. If you want to improve your skin, self-confidence, and self-esteem while bringing more positive thoughts into your life, you need to eliminate the toxins you accumulate throughout the day.

---

150 Professional requested not to disclose their name for personal reasons.

Essentially, this practitioner stresses that we must move our muscles and joints to healthily eliminate any toxic hormones before they linger in our bodies too long and make us sick. If we free our bodies from these toxins through the epidermis while working out, we are at the same time making our skin plumper, more vital, and more radiant. If not released, these toxins become stressors on the skin, and those toxic fluids will make you feel lethargic and fatigued, and therefore, less likely to believe in your inner beauty.

To work out your body is to take care of yourself and to love yourself, even if it's two to three times a week for thirty minutes. Believe in your value, believe in your body, believe in your beauty as a holistic composition and sweat out those toxins because that will allow you to really work what you have going for you on the inside to attain that glow.

I think that the "glow" hype is a subconscious search for inner beauty. The industry has just decided to call it "glow" because we love new fads. However, if you think about it, we cannot get this glow with a quick fix glow serum only. Although these products can be fantastic, they will only go so far. The real glow comes from within.

"Glow is the essence of beauty."

—ESTÉE LAUDER

AYURVEDA: AN OLD SCIENCE BECOMING THE "NEW SCIENCE"

Ayurveda is the mother of natural medicine. This philosophy understands nature and that we are all part of nature. Some people describe it as a guidebook for being in this universe. It explains how we coexist with our environment.

There exist three energies that govern everything called doshas, which you must understand in Ayurveda. Everything in the world is made up of these in different ratios: our bodies, our minds, your phone, this book, everything. The first is Vatta (airy, spacey, cold, dry, rough, anxious), the second is Pitta (hot, spreading, fiery, acidic, fast), and the third is Kapha (earth, water, damp, earthy, calm). They are just the colors red, yellow, blue, and they are in everything.[151]

Ayurveda is a term in Sanskrit meaning: Ayur (life) and Veda (knowledge), which translates to "knowledge of life" according to the National Ayurvedic Medical Association.[152] Since I began my research for this book, I was fascinated by the stories of people's lives changing for the better and particularly the tales of individuals being saved from chronic illness—diseases such as psoriasis, severe allergies, arthritis,

---

151 *The Beauty Closet* | Goop. 2019. *Goop*. Accessed October 6 2019. https://goop.com/beauty-closet-podcast/.

152 "What Is Ayurveda? — National Ayurvedic Medical Association." 2019. National Ayurvedic Medical Association. Accessed October 6 2019. https://www.ayurvedanama.org/what-is-ayurveda.

infertility, and more—with the help of Ayurveda. When one has chronic diseases, one is hindered from *feeling* beautiful. For this reason, it is important to look at beauty as something that begins with your internal health and well-being.

While we look at holistic and natural beauty working symbiotically with nature, Ayurveda has embodied this concept for about 5,000 years. Ayurvedic beliefs state that stress, unhealthy diet, the weather, and strained relationships with one's self or with others can misalign the balance that exists between a person's doshas.[153] According to the University of Maryland Medical Center, the result of unbalanced energies can make individuals more vulnerable to diseases and further unease. "The fundamental concept of Ayurveda is to maintain health. Ayurveda does not look at the disease. It looks at the host and an individual's vulnerability," according to Dr. Bala Manyam, a neurologist and professor emeritus at Southern Illinois University School of Medicine.[154] Many brands now see the effects of these practices and beliefs and are coming out with products with this same Ayurvedic philosophy, tackling the problem at its root.

---

153 Lallanilla, Marc. 2015. "Ayurveda: Facts About Ayurvedic Medicine." Livescience.Com. Accessed October 6 2019. https://www.livescience.com/42153-ayurveda.html#targetText=Ayurveda percent20is percent20an percent20ancient percent20health,) percent20and percent20veda percent20(knowledge.

154 Ibid.

Shadoh Punnapuzha[155] was born and raised in New York but lived and went to school in India for a few years. Shadoh's parents are from Kerala, India, one of the largest Ayurvedic hubs in the world, and she spent all of her summers there while growing up. On top of this, Shadoh's father had a background in botany, so Shadoh was always immersed in a culture of natural remedies. However, she did not embrace it when she was younger because it was the type of thing that your parents told you over and over again but you don't want to listen. However, one day, after she experienced a burnout in New York City while working for a Private Equity firm, she had no choice but to look in the direction of Ayurveda.

Shadoh shared with me her story into the Ayurvedic lifestyle to find her beauty.

> In my early thirties, I started getting eczema on my eyelids. I had high cystic acne and I also had all this other weird stuff I never experienced in my life before my burnout. I had to stop putting makeup on my eyelids because especially with eczema it just looked flakey. I was so frustrated because I was always interfacing with investors with the position I had at the PE firm I

---

155 Shadoh Punnapuzha is the Founder of Taïla Skincare. She is proving that when you combine the power of Ayurveda and science, you get divine results. After years of working at a PE firm in NYC and going through a burnout, Shadoh found her path to a healthy life and a healthy skin through Ayurveda.

worked for. I was dealing with a lot of very important people, and therefore how I put myself together was a big part of the job. I had no idea what to do.

I went to the dermatologist and he basically told me he did not know exactly what was happening to me, but the only way to really root it out was by stopping some of the skin care products I was using one by one. This would allow me to see which of them, if any, was causing these flares. Then in the meantime, he gave me a topical steroid to use. But I was not happy at all with the prescription.

I thought: *Really? That is just pacifying the symptoms!*

I cared about figuring out what was going on with me. I refused to take the treatment, but I started really digging for the root of my problem. One of the products I was using claimed it was "all natural" but eventually I found out it had synthetic preservatives in it.

Finally, I realized I had developed an allergic reaction to this synthetic preservative. Then on top of that, the dermatologist told me I was also having a reaction to sulfates in shampoos, which I had never had before. I was told that when you wash your hair, some of that shampoo goes on to your eyelids and then over time, this can build up an allergic reaction. But I didn't know if I wanted to believe all of this. After all, generations of today have the most increasing number of adult onset allergies than any other generations had before.

I didn't know what to use anymore because I didn't know how my skin would react to products. So, I ended up calling my father and he recommended to use natural oils.

This was the only thing that cured me. It was crazy. The only products that did not aggravate my skin were these natural oils. These were truly effective, safe, and natural.

After this, I was inspired, and I went on a trip to India to learn more about natural beauty and Ayurvedic approaches to beauty. I went back to Kerala to the birthplace of Ayurveda and properly learned not only the science but the lifestyle of Ayurveda.

While in India, I found my calling and created a team of Ayurvedic doctors to begin the formulation of Ayurvedic products. Then I came back to New York to figure out all the manufacturing, how to source and all these exchanges. I finally launched my brand

Taïla Skincare, a brand that combines the power of Ayurveda and science to provide incredible results.

The harsh reality is that often, even if we have the holistic and healthier option and path of life in front of us, we try to run off to the easy and quick fixes. In this case for Shadoh, it was the steroids. The reality is that we need to search for the origin of our problems and not only treat the symptoms in order to treat our internal beauty first and achieve a longer-lasting beauty. When our body is not satisfied inside, this shows on the outside. The real cure lies in a lifestyle change, not in a quick cream, pill, treatment, or surgery that will subside the external effects of unease.

AYURVEDIC INFLUENCE ON TODAY'S WELLNESS CRAZE

The Ayurvedic influence on holistic beauty and well-being is coming back at full force. As Jasmine Hemsley, a top food, health, and wellness expert, dives into the Goop Podcast, *Feeding your Digestive Fire,* these are some of the buzzwords in the holistic beauty and health sphere that are making lots of impact:[156]

---

156 "The Goop Podcast: Feeding Your Digestive Fire On Apple Podcasts." 2019. *Apple Podcasts.* Accessed November 4 2019. https://podcasts.apple.com/bs/podcast/feeding-your-digestive-fire/id1352546554?i=1000447315789.

- **Fermented foods:** include kimchi, sauerkraut, kefir, tempeh, kombucha, and yogurt. These foods may reduce heart disease risk while aiding digestion, immunity, and weight loss

- **Probiotics:** live bacteria and yeasts that are good for you, especially your digestive system. They are often called "good" or "helpful" bacteria because they help keep your gut healthy

- **Prebiotics:** types of dietary fiber that feed the friendly bacteria in your gut. This helps the gut bacteria produce nutrients for your colon cells and leads to a healthier digestive system

- **Massage:** rubbing and kneading of muscles and joints of the body with the hands, especially to relieve tension or pain

- **Reiki:** alleged to aid relaxation, assist in the body's natural healing processes, and develop emotional, mental, and spiritual well-being. It is also said to induce deep relaxation, help people cope with difficulties, relieve emotional stress, and improve overall well-being[157]

---

157 Newman, Tim, and OD Ann Marie Griff. 2017. "Reiki: What Is It And Are There Benefits?" Medical News Today. Accessed October 6 2019. https://www.medicalnewstoday.com/articles/308772.php.

- **Tongue cleaning:** scraping of the tongue with a tongue scraper, which can help remove its coating and prevent it from returning

- **Acupuncture:** a form of treatment that involves inserting very thin needles through a person's skin at specific points on the body, to various depths[158]

- **Oil pulling:** also known as "kavala" or "gundusha," an ancient Ayurvedic dental technique that involves swishing a tablespoon of oil in your mouth on an empty stomach for around twenty minutes. This action supposedly draws out toxins in your body, primarily to improve oral health but also to improve your overall health[159]

- **Pranayama:** a practice relating to the control and regulation of the breath through specific breathing techniques and exercises. It can help clear physical and emotional blocks or obstacles in the body so that the breath, and prana, can flow freely[160]

---

158 Brazier, Yvette, and MS Yamini Ranchod. 2017. "Acupuncture: How It Works, Uses, Benefits, And Risks." Medical News Today. Accessed October 6 2019. https://www.medicalnewstoday.com/articles/156488.php.

159 "I Tried Oil Pulling For (Almost) A Week: Here's What Happened." 2019. Fashionista. Accessed October 6 2019. https://fashionista.com/2014/03/oil-pulling.

160 "Pranayama | Ekhart Yoga." 2019. *Ekhartyoga.Com.* Accessed October 6 2019. https://www.ekhartyoga.com/resources/styles/pranayama.

- **Yoga:** a group of physical, mental, and spiritual practices or disciplines that originated in ancient India. This can increase flexibility, increase muscle strength and tone, improve respiration, energy and vitality, help maintain a balanced metabolism, weight reduction, help cardio and circulatory health, improve athletic performance, protect from injury, and more[161]

"All these terms and trends we are experiencing are Ayurveda and have been a way of life for a long time. In Eastern cultures we are only beginning to adapt these on an individual basis in order to capitalize on the branding. All of these are techniques and they all need to be done correctly and in the proper doses,"[162] Jasmine Hemsley says.

We are beginning to understand more and more how much the gut affects the mind and emotions. Although in Western cultures we might think these are part of a new science or cutting-edge research, these terms listed above have been more recently adopted from old traditional Eastern medicines and sciences such as Ayurveda.

---

161 "Benefits of Yoga | American Osteopathic Association." 2019. *American Osteopathic Association.* Accessed October 6 2019. https://osteopathic.org/what-is-osteopathic-medicine/benefits-of-yoga/.

162 "The Goop Podcast: Feeding Your Digestive Fire On Apple Podcasts." 2019. *Apple Podcasts.* Accessed November 4 2019. https://podcasts.apple.com/bs/podcast/feeding-your-digestive-fire/id1352546554?i=1000447315789.

HEALTHY COMPLEXION OF THE SKIN

A clean canvas, as Peter Thomas Roth[163] calls it, is when the skin is perfectly cleansed and exfoliated. When we have a clean canvas, we can have the liberty to express our beauty in any way we want. Makeup or no makeup, we can *feel* beautiful.

Peter says, "If you have a cleansed and exfoliated canvas, your skin care treatments and products will work better, and your skin will look better, so you can go with no makeup or less."

Everyone has their way of showing their beauty. Dr. Barbara Sturm[164] states, "I don't want to hide my face with foundation. I want it to look real, dewy, and glowing."

PRACTICING SAFE BEAUTY

Before, no one thought about the possibility of personal care potentially being unsafe, but now everybody is thinking

---

163 Peter Thomas Roth is the CEO, founder, and formulator of Peter Thomas Roth Clinical Skin Care, is an influential segment leader in the beauty industry and continues to corner the clinical market as a groundbreaking, results-focused innovator. Today, Peter's comprehensive range of products are sold worldwide in over eighty countries, with Peter leading all research and development efforts at his state-of-the-art lab and manufacturing facility.

164 Dr. Barbara Sturm is the founder and CEO of Dr. Barbara Sturm Molecular Cosmetics. She is a German aesthetics doctor, widely renowned for her anti-inflammatory philosophy and her non-surgical anti-aging skin treatments. Dr. Sturm translated science from her clinical research and orthopedic practice into the field of aesthetics and has been a success ever since.

about it. Miranda Kerr describes it in *The Beauty Closet* podcast in the following way, "It is important people know what you are putting on your body because your body is a vessel that is constantly filling up and you need to fill it up with safe, clean products."[165]

Nneka Leiba[166] says on *The Beauty Closet* podcast by Goop, "It's crazy that when you go buy a product that is essentially going to be making you *feel* more beautiful, the last thing you want to be worrying about is the negative effects it will have on your health."[167] Companies are changing now, and consumers are starting to have much higher expectations. Now consumers are less willing to invest in harmful products, but it is not so trivial to know how harmful a product is. Until companies and brands are fully transparent with consumers, we need to know who we can trust and what red flags to look out for.[168]

These are a few websites/apps to find out the safety "cleanliness" of a product:

---

165 *The Beauty Closet* | Goop. 2019. *Goop.* Accessed October 6 2019. https://goop.com/beauty-closet-podcast/.

166 Nneka Leiba is the Vice President of EWG's Healthy Living Science and leads the team to translate complicated scientific topics, particularly ones dealing with the effects of everyday chemical exposures on our health, into easily accessible tips and advice.

167 "Why Are There Still Toxic Ingredients In Beauty Products? | Goop." 2019. *Goop.* Accessed October 6 2019. https://goop.com/beauty-closet-podcast/why-are-there-still-toxic-ingredients-in-beauty-products/.

168 Ibid.

- Think Dirty
- GoodGuide
- CosmeEthics
- EWG Skin Deep
- Detox Me
- Dirty Dozen

Look up products yourself and make sure the products you are investing in rank as safe or clean products by the afore-mentioned platforms. Buzz words such as "all-natural" or "organic" nowadays mean little to nothing, especially in the US where the beauty and skin care safety regulations are not as tight as the EU for example. Think about it this way. Poison ivy is natural and organic… will you put that on your face or body? Since the usage of such words on product packaging are not always regulated, it is hard to make educated purchasing choices, especially because the consumer feels like they are being informed with these words, but in reality, they are being misled.[169]

Although it's shocking that in this day and age beauty companies are still using toxic ingredients in their formulas, it is happening everywhere. Hence, it is important to go the extra

---

169 "These 5 Apps Tell You What's In Your Beauty Products So You Can Shop Safer." 2019. Bustle. Accessed October 6 2019. https://www.bustle.com/p/5-apps-that-tell-you-whats-in-beauty-products-because-knowledge-is-power-11997650.

mile in understanding the ingredients in the products you use. I hope that there will soon be a better way to regulate and rank these products on an objective standard to make the lives of consumers easier.

A good fact to remember is that, "Most people use 126 ingredients on their skin daily, and shockingly, nearly eighty-five percent of the ingredients approved by the Food and Drug Administration for use in personal care products have not been evaluated for safety by the agency, the industry's Cosmetics Ingredient Review panel, or any other regulatory body."[170]

This is frightening.

I believe people are getting tired of these marketing schemes and want to seek the truth. As consumers get more informed, *faux marketing* will become even more recognizable and disregarded. I believe in the years to come consumers will focus on effectiveness, quality, and safety before they look at the appeal of the product's advertisement.

Greenwashing, the practice of making an unsubstantiated or misleading claim about the environmental benefits of a

---

170 "7 Apps To Help You Check For Chemicals & Find Non-Toxic Alternatives." 2019. Tox Free Family. Accessed October 6 2019. https://toxfreefamily.com/mobile-apps-to-reduce-harsh-chemical-exposure/.

product, service, technology or company practice,[171] is a new fad that has made conscious consumers of today reluctant to believe in what a brand claims of their product. Hence, this trend must come to an end if the beauty industry wants to earn a positive and trustworthy relationship with its consumer base.

After all, the beauty industry would benefit enormously from making consumers feel reassured that the products they purchase will enhance the way they feel, rather than have them worry about whether or not the products are toxic for their bodies.

CAUTION: *GREENWASHING*

"According to the 2017 Green Beauty Barometer survey results, seventy-four percent of women with children at home, and sixty percent of women without kids at home, claim that purchasing green or natural beauty products was important to them."[172] These numbers are staggering, considering that the indications of "green" products are a lot of times not being regulated.

171 "What Is Greenwashing?—Definition From Whatis.Com." 2019. Whatis.Com. Accessed October 6 2019. https://whatis. techtarget.com/definition/greenwashing.

172 "THE GREEN BAROMETER SURVEY." 2019. *Kari Gran Skin Care*. Accessed October 6 2019. https://karigran.com/pages/ the-green-barometer-survey.

People don't really think about what "green" actually means. They just think, "It must be good for me." But just because something has natural ingredients doesn't necessarily mean that it's safe or that it's in alignment with your skin's needs.

When someone talks about "organic," and "natural," "clean," or "green" beauty, what does that even mean?

"Greenwashing is when a company uses words or images to make a product seem more natural or non-toxic than it actually is. The words "clean," "organic," and "natural" are being thrown around for consumers to be attracted to certain products," Arden Martin explains.[173]

The word "clean" at the moment has all the hype. Clean just means the product is safe for your skin, not that all the ingredients are natural or organic. Companies, however, use "clean" in whatever way they want, as Dr. Sturm points out.[174]

---

173 Arden Martin is a teacher of Vedic Meditation and co-founder of The Spring Meditation Studio in New York City. She cares deeply about bringing more transparency to the US personal care industry and works with Beautycounter to educate people about what "clean beauty" really means.

174 Dr. Barbara Sturm is the founder and CEO of Dr. Barbara Sturm Molecular Cosmetics. She is a German aesthetics doctor, widely renowned for her anti-inflammatory philosophy and her non-surgical anti-aging skin treatments. Dr. Sturm translated science from her clinical research and orthopedic practice into the field of aesthetics and has been a success ever since.

Behind a "clean" foundation product, as Arden shows in one of her stories on Instagram, it can say, "Manufacturers, suppliers, and others provide what you see on here, and we have not verified it." Then when looking at the ingredients of this product, Arden shows the first ingredient being water, which immediately means the product needs preservatives to prevent mold. In this case not all preservatives are bad. Some are safe and are needed to keep the shelf life of a product. There are safe and unsafe preservatives, but this "clean" product Arden exhibited did not have safe ones. Instead it had Methylparaben and Propylparaben, which should be avoided if you want to be conscious about maintaining your reproductive health. These types of parabens are hormone disruptors.[175] Further, Arden points out that fragrance on the ingredients section is a red flag, as it is an unknown in terms of what is in it. This "ingredient" can contain hormone disruptors too, and it has been linked to allergies, neurotoxicity, and other complications.

According to Arden there is no way of knowing what is in a given fragrance because there could be up to 3,000 formulations of chemicals to form that fragrance. She therefore advises people to stick people to companies that don't

---

175 Arden Martin is a teacher of Vedic Meditation and co-founder of The Spring Meditation Studio in New York City. She cares deeply about bringing more transparency to the US personal care industry and works with Beautycounter to educate people about what "clean beauty" really means.

mention the word fragrance as an ingredient at the back of the product but rather list the breakdown of what ingredients make up the scent. Sometimes these products don't even need to be fragranced. If you see the word "clean" on anything insinuating that the product is fresh, or clean, or natural, or safe, make no assumptions that this is true and research it.

There is also a loophole in personal care legislation in the US, where companies tweak their ingredients in secret and call it a "trade secret." Just like the use of the word "fragrance," we don't know what chemicals are in that "trade secret." For anyone who wants to get better about using clean products, I recommend going with companies that are very transparent, disclose all their ingredients, and provide a channel for consumers to raise questions.

Not all chemicals are bad. We should not be afraid of the word chemical. We just need to know if the chemicals being used are safe. Safe chemicals can actually enhance the potency of your skin care without having to make them harmful for your skin. It's really about the quality and function, as not all chemicals are created equally.

For those worried about the potency of products, one alternative of these that Arden used is "safer synthetic" ingredients that are safe yet potent. Bakuchiol, for example, is the safer version of Retinol, she says. Retinol is commonly prescribed by dermatologists and you can find Retinol or vitamin A derivative ingredients in a lot of skin care. It's meant to be an anti-aging ingredient and a cell regenerator. But as it is commonly known, the issue with Retinol is it can lead to increased irritation and create sensitivity in the skin. It can also increase your sensitivity to the sun. Arden referenced a 2014 study that shows Bakuchiol, traditionally used in Chinese Traditional Medicine and Ayurveda, produces the same or very similar results as Retinol when used on the skin. Beautycounter[176] discovered this study, and they started to compare Bakuchiol's results to Retinol's results. They found that they were very similar, so they developed this skin care line using Bakuchiol as the main ingredient as a safer Retinol alternative.

Arden's passion for health and well-being started like this:

> It really started with my own meditation practice because it was the most transformative thing for my inner sense of happiness. It was transformative for my confidence. As a woman growing up in mainstream society, beauty has always been on my mind. I always wanted to be beautiful and I was always comparing myself to other women, as so many of

---

176 Beautycounter is an American Direct Retail skin care and cosmetics brand that as of 2018 has been at the forefront of this movement of clean beauty but also high performing.

us do. I also carried a lot of insecurity and lacked confidence for most of my life.

I found that with meditation, a lot of that insecurity and a lot of those feelings I had about myself started to shift. My confidence completely transformed with a regular meditation practice. I started to tap into this sense of self-love I didn't even know was possible. And right around the time I started to feel much more confident in myself and love for myself, I started to have people telling me I was glowing. That my skin looked amazing. That I looked beautiful.

We joke in the meditation community that; you get that glow from meditating. What that really means is that you're not stressed out, you know when you're feeling well, and you're not anxious. As a result, you are smiling more often than not!

Stress affects your hormones and hormones affect your skin. It really all comes down to your stress and your mental state. All of this has a real effect on your outer appearance and what's perceived as your outer beauty.

At first, I felt like I didn't really have a clear direction. But, for me, meditation has really had a direct correlation with enhancement on my outer beauty.

BE CONSCIOUS OF WHAT YOU ARE PUTTING ON YOUR SKIN

Pregnancy—we see all this fear of what we put on our skin during pregnancy, and it has been hard for women to have a relationship with skin care and makeup because of the ambiguities in the safety of even the products that claim to be safe.

I love the approach Stephanie Peterson[177] takes toward her beauty brand, Smoothie Beauty. Stephanie's mission is making smoothies for your face with the idea of using toxic-free edible ingredients in her skin care to reduce an absorption of about 1,512 unsafe chemicals per person a year. As she says, "The proof is in the pudding."

Stephanie's products for this reason are great for pregnant and breastfeeding mothers and teenage girls who need to be careful about using anything that will disrupt their hormones. She explains that pregnant mothers are starting to

---

177 Stephanie Peterson is a model and the founder of Smoothie Beauty, a clean and organic skin care line that is truly fresh without any toxic chemicals, additives, or preservatives. She is also the creator of The Global Beauty blog. She has modeled in more than fifteen countries, with the likes of Clinique, Mary Kay and Pandora, among others.

understand how our skin absorbs these toxic chemicals and are hyper aware of this while breastfeeding and general pregnancy prep. More and more I see a trend where people are beginning to want to use ingredients on their skin that would be safe to eat.

Get Smart About Ingredients

As early as the 1950s, entrepreneurs like Jacques Courtin-Clarins and Yves Rocher began to experiment making cosmetics from plants rather than chemicals, decades ahead of perceived demand. They, and their counterparts in other industries such as food and cleaning materials who talked about the dangers of chemical ingredients and the need for environmental sustainability, were often dismissed as crazy, or at best irrelevant. Today, many of their ideas are mainstream.

—GEOFFREY JONES[178]

As Geoffrey explains, these ideas now are present in our daily interactions with beauty products. This is one of the most amazing trends that could be happening to the industry

---

178 Geoffrey Jones is the Isidor Straus Professor of Business History, and Faculty Chair of the School's Business History Initiative in the Harvard Business School.

because as more consumers become aware of the importance of ingredients and their safety, more competition between brands will occur, giving clients safer options to choose from. However, we need to be careful because this competition is also pushing for a lot of *faux marketing.*

Speaking about this subject with Dr. Sturm, she said, "There is a big movement around clean beauty, non-toxic, organic or natural. But clean and organic beauty has a different definition in different countries and in different companies. It is essential to know all of this because some countries consider some pesticides as organic." Dr. Sturm further highlighted that natural products can be crucial to wellness and health, but not all. For example, manchineel, stinging nettle (depending on how you consume it), hogweed, and poison ivy amongst others can be unsafe in the long run.

Dr. Sturm champions natural products because she believes the best and most effective ingredients usually come from nature. She says, "My natural ingredients are tested for safety and then they are synthesized to get rid of all the allergens. This way we can make sure the ingredients are pure and consistent." Dr. Sturm likes to use natural ingredients as well as lab-made ingredients, but she again stresses the importance of understanding that just because it is made in a lab does not mean it is bad for you, as we hear from Arden Martin above.

Dr. Sturm's focus on efficacy, science, and safety make her products so effective and ultimately, so popular.

Although it is not widely known, clean ingredients can also be very high-performing. We do not have to sacrifice performance in order to have clean products. Don't be afraid of chemicals in your skin care and don't be afraid of preservatives. They're actually important for the shelf life and effectiveness of your skin care. As Arden stressed, "If you know the product contains water, you don't want it to grow mold, so you want preservatives, clean ones of course, but you need them. It's really all about the safety of the ingredients, how well those ingredients will be held in storage, and how rigorously the ingredients and formulations have been tested."

It's really not about buying products that are 100 percent natural or plant based. It is about how committed the company or brand is to the safety and efficacy of their products.

Peter Thomas Roth's HOT Ingredient List:

1. **SPF Sunscreen**

2. **Retinol:** An anti-aging powerhouse ingredient that visibly helps improve the look of fine lines, wrinkles, uneven skin tone, texture and radiance. Peter uses a unique, pure

and potent solution of Time-Released Microencapsulated Retinol that delivers a gradual stream of non-irritating Retinol all night long while you sleep.

3. **Hyaluronic Acid:** A potent hydrator that can attract and retain up to 1,000 times its weight in water from moisture in the atmosphere. This is the hero ingredient in Peter Thomas Roth's cult-favorite Water Drench® Hyaluronic Cloud Cream, which is packed with a 30 percent Hyaluronic Acid Complex that moisturizes skin with a liquid cloud of pure water vapor.

4. **Peptides:** Peptides in your skin send a signal to produce new collagen, leading to the appearance of younger, more supple-looking skin. Applying topical treatments with peptides can help skin appear younger by visibly reducing the look of fine lines and wrinkles. Peptides are a key ingredient in Peter Thomas Roth's Peptide 21™ Wrinkle Resist Serum and Peptide 21™ Lift & Firm Moisturizer.

5. **Neuropeptides:** Neuropeptides are communicators, just like Peptides. Unlike Peptides, however, Neuropeptides in the body interact with neurons to help keep the skin's surface appearing relaxed and youthful. Applying topical treatments with Neuropeptides can help reduce the look of expression lines. Neuropeptides

are a key ingredient in Peter Thomas Roth's Peptide 21™ Wrinkle Resist Serum and Peptide 21™ Lift & Firm Moisturizer.

6. **Glycolic Acid:** An Alpha Hydroxy Acid (AHA) that works as a chemical exfoliator to help improve the look of pores, smoothness, brightness and clarity while reducing the look of fine lines, wrinkles and uneven skin tone. Peter says Glycolic Acid is an amazing ingredient because it's generally well tolerated by all skin types.

7. **Pumpkin Enzymes:** A gentle-yet-effective exfoliant that helps dissolve dead skin cells and remove surface impurities to uncover a smoother, younger, brighter-looking complexion. Pumpkin Enzyme is the hero ingredient of Peter Thomas Roth's Pumpkin Enzyme Mask Enzymatic Dermal Resurfacer.

8. **Salicylic Acid:** Peter Thomas Roth says this ingredient is not only great for acne, which is what people tend to use Salicylic Acid for, but also great for helping to reduce the appearance of wrinkles. You can find this ingredient in his acne products as well as many of his anti-aging products, including Anti-Aging Cleansing Gel, Peptide 21™ Amino Acid Exfoliating Peel Pads and more.

Maria Calderon The Newest Ingredients:

1. **Fermented extracts**

2. **Prebiotics:** Present a double activity allowing the sustainable and ecological Ecoflora of skin and hair ecosystem.

3. **Human Growth Factors:** Participate in the proliferation processes, differentiation, maintenance of skin homeostasis and in healing. It acts both in the morphogenesis of the follicle during the embryonic stage and in its development during adulthood, favoring growth in the different cycles of hair regeneration.

4. **Natural Biopolymers:** Environmental pollution and sunlight are considered the main causes of premature extrinsic aging. Natural biopolymers form a resistant, flexible and non-occlusive film on the skin that acts as a natural barrier against harmful exogenous agents.

Dr. Ava Shamban's Top Effectiveness Ingredient Picks:

1. **SPF Sunscreen**

2. **Salicylic Acid:** Causes shedding of the outer layer of skin.

3. **Hyaluronic Acid:** Binds to water to help retain moisture and can reduce wrinkles, redness and dermatitis.

4. **Retinoids:** The most used and most studied anti-aging compounds—reduce fine lines and wrinkles by increasing the production of collagen.

COLLAGEN—THE HOT TOPIC

In 2018 Americans spent 4.3 billion dollars on Collagen products,[179] but were they all getting their money's worth?[180]

Maria Calderon,[181] who is a chemical cosmetic pharmaceutical specialist can better elaborate.

Collagen is the most abundant protein in your body, and it is what keeps skin firm and your joints, tendons, and muscles together. Many are desperately

---

179 WIRE, BUSINESS. 2019. "Global $4.6 Billion Collagen Market by Product Type, Source, Application and Region—Forecast To 2023—Researchandmarkets.Com." *Businesswire.Com.* Accessed October 6 2019. https://www.businesswire.com/news/home/20190308005227/en/Global-4.6-Billion-Collagen-Market-Product-Type.

180 Ibid.

181 Maria Calderon is the CEO and founder of Kosmetai, founder of Institut Nahia, and founder of Juveskin, S.L. company, where she serves as Director General and is the Technical Director of PRODUCTOS BIORGANICOS, S.L. Maria is a chemical cosmetic pharmaceutical specialist and licensed expert in the evaluation of the security and information files of cosmetic products.

trying to improve their skin by topically applying or ingesting collagen products because as we age our rate of production of collagen is reduced significantly, allowing not only the production of wrinkles on our skin but other internal wear and tear.

Now it seems that collagen has become a buzzword that makes consumers want to buy products that contain this protein. However, some products that are not of great quality put collagen in its regular form, and in this form the molecule is too heavy to penetrate to the deeper layers of the skin, where the collagen production is focused. What is happening now is that people are paying for collagen for it to sit on top of their skin with no effect or potency—no matter high or low percentage of collagen.

Collagen must be hydrolyzed, so the molecules can be absorbed. Hydrolysis converts collagen into smaller molecules. One should apply this collagen topically for the maximum effect and the best use of your investment.

Studies show that hydrolyzed correctly collagen can be effectively absorbed at the topical level. For oral collagen however, there is currently no scientific study conducted by the FDA or the MA that proves stomach or intestinal acid don't disintegrate the collagen protein when ingested in its powdered or liquid form before it reaches the moment of absorption. We will have to wait for further research.

HUGE "NO-NOS"

Nneka Leiba[182] strongly recommends that you reject any product that contains any of the following:

1. **Carbon Black:** used in some mascaras and is known to be a carcinogen
2. **Formaldehyde:** some Keratin products contain this, and it is a well-known carcinogen
3. **Mercury:** potent neurotoxin. A lot of people take care of the amount of mercury intake with fish, but makeup has it too.
   a. It is known to damage your brain and the development of a fetus
   b. It is sometimes used as a preservative in some eye makeup products and whitening creams

---

182 Nneka Leiba is the Vice President of EWG's Healthy Living Science and leads the team to translate complicated scientific topics, particularly ones dealing with the effects of everyday chemical exposures on our health, into easily accessible tips and advice.

Many more have been predicted to be toxic but given the sheer number of ingredients in the market, in-depth studies can be very time consuming.

You might be thinking: "Well everyone says everything gives you cancer nowadays so what does it even matter?"

The problem is that we don't just put one bad chemical on our bodies at a time. We are being exposed to a huge load of harmful chemicals in most of our skin care, makeup, and hair care. That, all together, can make up for a big yearly dose of toxic intake. These may also cause reactions with each other inside your body and may tamper with your health. "Some of these are also active in low levels and they affect us biologically in small doses. They specifically disrupt our endocrine system,"[183] Nneka Leiba says on *The Beauty Closet* podcast by Goop.[184]

Further underlining this, Carol Kwiatkowski[185] says to *The Guardian*:

183 "Why Are There Still Toxic Ingredients In Beauty Products? | Goop." 2019. *Goop*. Accessed October 6 2019. https://goop.com/beauty-closet-podcast/why-are-there-still-toxic-ingredients-in-beauty-products/.

184 Ibid.

185 Carol Kwiatkowski is the Executive Director of The Endocrine Disruption Exchange (*TEDx*), a not-for-profit research foundation focused on reducing harmful chemicals in the environment.

If you think about the chronic conditions the world is experiencing now—like fertility problems, thyroid conditions, diabetes, ADHD—these are all heavily impacted by hormones. Prevalence rates are sky-rocketing. We just don't know what is causing it. It's undeniable that environmental chemicals are part of the picture. And we just continue to ignore them.[186]

ABOUT FDA LEGISLATION

FDA Regulations surrounding personal care products have not been updated since 1938. [187]

I know what you're thinking: *Ummmm, what?*

The craziest part is that since then "about 100,000 chemicals have been brought to market since," says Nneka Leiba on *The Beauty Closet* by Goop podcast.[188]

186 Zanolli, Lauren. 2019. "Pretty Hurts: Are Chemicals In Beauty Products Making Us Ill?." *The Guardian*. Accessed October 6 2019. https://www.theguardian.com/us-news/2019/may/23/are-chemicals-in-beauty-products-making-us-ill.

187 "FDA Authority Over Cosmetics: How Cosmetics Are Not FDA-Approved." 2019. *U.S. Food And Drug Administration*. Accessed October 6 2019. https://www.fda.gov/cosmetics/cosmetics-laws-regulations/fda-authority-over-cosmetics-how-cosmetics-are-not-fda-approved-are-fda-regulated.

188 "Why Are There Still Toxic Ingredients in Beauty Products? | Goop." 2019. *Goop*. Accessed October 6 2019. https://goop.com/beauty-closet-podcast/why-are-there-still-toxic-ingredients-in-beauty-products/.

According to the FDA's website:

"The law does not require cosmetic products and ingredients, other than color additives, to have FDA approval before they go on the market." [189]

"In the United States, federal laws are enacted by Congress, and the Congress authorizes certain government agencies like the FDA meaning that change in FDA's legal authority over cosmetics would require Congress to change the law." [190]

FDA states that the safety of a product can be adequately evidenced through:

a. "Reliance on already available toxicological test data on individual ingredients and product formulations that are similar in composition to the particular cosmetic." [191]

b. "Performance of any additional toxicological and other tests that are appropriate in light of such existing data and information." [192]

---

189 "FDA Authority Over Cosmetics: How Cosmetics Are Not FDA-Approved." 2019. *U.S. Food And Drug Administration.* Accessed October 6 2019. https://www.fda.gov/cosmetics/cosmetics-laws-regulations/fda-authority-over-cosmetics-how-cosmetics-are-not-fda-approved-are-fda-regulated.

190 Ibid.

191 Ibid.

192 Ibid.

If The Personal Care Products Safety Act, which would modernize how the FDA currently regulates personal care products, becomes a law it would require manufacturers to prove their products and ingredients are safe before they go out onto the market. Although we would hope this was the case already, it's not. [193]

Nneka explains further on the *The Beauty Closet* by Goop podcast why this Safety Act has not passed yet. She says, "The reason is that on Capitol Hill, nothing happens in the sphere of personal care because of opposition. For many years, there was a lot of money in the opposition. The good thing about the Personal Care Product Safety Act is that there are a lot of companies that support it."[194] Now, it is much more common to support this bill because it is becoming such an apparent conversation in the beauty sector, whereas people before weren't aware of the issue, as Ewelina Aiossa[195] mentioned to me. With many companies on board there is hope for

---

193 "The Personal Care Product Safety Act." 2019. EWG. Accessed November 4 2019. https://www.ewg.org/personalcareproductsafetyact.

194 "Why Are There Still Toxic Ingredients in Beauty Products? | Goop." 2019. *Goop*. Accessed October 6 2019. https://goop.com/beauty-closet-podcast/why-are-there-still-toxic-ingredients-in-beauty-products/.

195 Ewelina Aiossa is the Assistant Vice President of Marketing at SkinCeuticals, L'Oreal. She serves on UBM—Dermatology Times Industry Council and SkinCeuticals (SC) Leadership Team panel. She has a strong knowledge of the aesthetic business, professional channel, products, and ingredients.

regulations in the US to become tighter and for our products to be safer for consumers.

If this bill were to be passed, it would give the FDA the authority to adequately police the beauty care space. At the moment, the FDA cannot mandate a recall even if a product has been shown to be toxic or unsafe for human use. In addition, the FDA would be required to review a handful of chemicals every year to ensure that the latest scientific research is available for all of them.[196]

"We are so behind the EU and other countries. The EU bans and restricts about 1,400 chemicals in the personal care sector and the US bans or restricts fewer than ten. We, Environmental Working Group,[197] use literature and the regulations from the EU, Canada, Japan, and other Asian countries because they have more research and more regulation for personal care products," says Nneka.[198]

---

196 "Why Are There Still Toxic Ingredients in Beauty Products? | Goop." 2019. *Goop.* Accessed October 6 2019. https://goop.com/beauty-closet-podcast/why-are-there-still-toxic-ingredients-in-beauty-products/.

197 The Environmental Working Group's mission is to empower people to live healthier lives in a healthier environment. With breakthrough research and education, we drive consumer choice and civic action.

198 "Why Are There Still Toxic Ingredients in Beauty Products? | Goop." 2019. *Goop.* Accessed October 6 2019. https://goop.com/beauty-closet-podcast/why-are-there-still-toxic-ingredients-in-beauty-products/.

Innocent Until Proven Guilty:

The US allows all products out to the market until proven to be unsafe. You could bring a product to market, having absolutely no study or quality system of manufacturing practices, and still sell it. On the contrary, Europe, South Korea, and Japan do not release anything to market before it has been proven to be safe.

Maria Calderon explains that Europe is a pioneer in everything that is regulated for the approval of ingredients to be put out in the market. Not only are they pioneers, but also EU member countries have created a mandatory cosmetovigilance system.[199]

DO SOME DIGGING

Maria mentions that the world of cosmetics is lacking in giving information to consumers for why some formulations are done one way or another. Therefore, the power to make an educated decision on the type of skin care or makeup to purchase is not given to consumers. It's a blind shot.

Maria provides the following example with foundation:

---

199 A cosmetovigilance system is the ongoing and systematic monitoring of the safety of cosmetics in terms of human health. The aim is to detect adverse effects of cosmetic products and to prevent adverse effects by taking appropriate measures.

When a consumer goes to buy a foundation, they don't know if that foundation is going to clog their pores or not. They don't know if they should be using a foundation, or maybe a BB cream instead. They don't know if a certain formulation in a foundation is going to cause a dependence for that product. They don't know if that foundation has an active ingredient that will make their skin create some type of irritation or inflammation. We are filled with unknowns.

In other words, a consumer cannot ask for a salad with tomatoes and peppers because they don't know what a tomato or pepper is. Therefore, it is critical to choose a brand you trust will know what you need in your salad and take it upon themselves to explain why the ingredients in your salad are the best for YOU. Essentially, as a consumer you must look for a brand that tells you what the ingredients are and what they do. Find a brand that bets on the results and advises on a person-by-person basis.

I know this is a lot of information. There is no need to go into immediate panic mode! The good news is that skin care is used in small doses, so it is not too late to become a conscious consumer now. Better late than never, as they say.

Start being a smarter beauty consumer and dig deeper into ingredients and their formulations when you purchase products. In chapter 10, you will see many tips and recommendations from professionals that will help you make more informed choices.

CHAPTER 6

INFLUENCED TO BE A "HACKABLE HUMAN"

——

TWO SIDES TO EVERY COIN

All technological advancements in the world have positive and negative aspects.

When I was young, the argument was whether having a cell phone was good or bad for a ten-year-old kid? I remember hearing all sorts of responses to this from my friends' parents.

My mother saw more positives than negatives to this device. She found that being able to contact me at all times and vice versa carried more weight than the harm of me texting my friends all day, which I kind of did. Other mothers though, believed the negative consequences of giving a child a cell phone would have them become "addicted" and that outweighed the positive aspects. Many of my friends therefore did not have phones until an older age.

While there is nothing wrong with either of these thought processes, I am one to always use the new technology that is available to me in hopes of good outcomes. We are currently living in the twenty-first century, where every day countless individuals work hard on technological advancements to make our daily activities easier, faster, better or simply more interesting. *So, why not take advantage of this?*

For the consumers of the beauty industry to benefit from these advancements, there needs to be a strong sense of inner beauty cultivated. What I call inner beauty, others may call confidence, physical and mental health, self-acceptance, self-esteem, self-love, etc. Ultimately, these are one and the same.

Unfortunately, we live in a time when many people are less comfortable *feeling* beautiful due to the accessibility of so much visual content by which to compare ourselves constantly. This is not only happening with millennials and Generation Zers, but also with Generation Xers and Boomers, who are constantly reminded that youth is the icon of beauty, and in consequence, not them.

At the same time, I believe there are just as many reasons to *feel* even more empowered and more beautiful with social media. For the first time in history we can effortlessly see the many images and perceptions of beauty in the world by simply scrolling and clicking. It's almost miraculous we can *see* what is out there just like that. Without leaving your bedroom you can see people from different backgrounds, people expressing themselves, people living their lives, and people who have other perceptions of beauty than you do.

Although social media does not always portray the truth, we can at least get a glimpse of what is out there. If you have the opportunity to travel, do so. Travel allows us to perceive better and live an experience that reframes our perception of beauty better than any digital or virtual experience.

OPENING OUR MINDS

Only when we have seen can we truly cultivate our own inner beauty, value what we have, and value our differences.

Regarding this, Chinwe Esimai says: [200]

---

200 Chinwe Esimai is the Managing Director and Chief Anti-Bribery Officer at Citigroup, Inc. She is also an award-winning lawyer, author, and speaker who is passionate about inspiring generations of immigrant women leaders.

A lot of change still needs to take place, but we are moving in the right direction. In general, social media has created opportunities for people to brand themselves and have a voice. This sort of individual expression is also indicative of one's beauty. Through social media, societies' perception and understanding of beauty is becoming broader, as people are exposed to others who are far from anyone they have seen in their immediate environments—people who have radically different standards and expressions of beauty.

On the same note, Bisila Bokoko[201] shared a similar point of view to Chinwe. Bisila battled with finding herself beautiful, growing up in Spain as a native black African. Social media for her was an outlet to see beautiful people out there who did look like her, as she didn't see many around her growing up. She says:

Technology is democratizing beauty because beauty is everywhere. It has enhanced the ability to feel beautiful. Before, beauty was a concept that separated us from each other, and thanks to social media

---

201 Bisila Bokoko is the founder and CEO of BBES, a business development agency in New York that represents and promotes international market brands. She has inspired thousands of people and organizations around the world through conferences in which she has motivated others to pursue dreams, think big, and talk about empowerment, entrepreneurship, geopolitics, and personal branding.

creating window to the world, I think we have a more unified concept of beauty around the world.

Now, we see that a transgender can be beautiful, people from all different races can be beautiful, people with vitiligo can be beautiful, albino people can be beautiful. The thing is that it is hard to imagine something we cannot see. This visual content allows us to see and therefore understand.

We are getting more used to this beauty from exposure to visual content. Before, carefully handpicked photographs in magazines dictated what beauty had to look like. Now with social media and technology we can see a lot more people who look like us and like all diversity of people.

We can now imitate or want to look like any type of influencers because we all still love having an example to follow. We no longer have to be frustrated by the fact that we will never look like people in the magazines—something I struggled with as a little girl.

Also, now, if you don't like to wear makeup and you rock your bare skin with confidence, no one will criticize you. On the contrary, most people would admire you. If you like to wear a cake of makeup, people applaud you as well! Both of these extremes and everyone in between can be beautiful, and this is a concept that began mainly with influencers, and You-tubers, showing you how they do beauty at home—that it was not up to the makeup artist only to make you *feel* beautiful. YouTube actually has so much impact on the beauty industry. The beauty industry revolution happened by showing people they could do it at home.

When it comes to Instagram, I believe you have the possibility of posting and *feeling* beautiful with what you post. Before when you had a great photo of yourself, the most you could do was hang it around your home. Now we can all feel like the celebrities of our own lives and that is something very powerful.

But of course, like everything, there is also a negative side to technology because we get carried away and give too much power to the validation of others. It is all about the mindset you have. You have the choice to choose technology and social media for confidence and empowerment, and not to compare and create insecurities.

I believe social media is a beautiful tool to make the world a more inclusive place.

It's not all a fairytale. The same social networks that can make us discover and learn can also make us slaves to the content we see. However, if we are conscious about the way we consume content, it is a treasure to explore. It is almost as if you have to prepare your guard to dive into the never-ending beauty content out there.

DIGITAL DICTATORSHIP

As Yuval Noah Harari, the author of *21st Lessons for the 21st Century,* or more widely known as the author of *Sapiens* says:

"It is not about the technology itself; technology can be built to create something wonderful or it can be the basis for the rise of a digital dictatorship."[202]

It is up to us to decide if we are going to allow social media, influencers, and the world of digital advertising to be a digital dictatorship.

We need to have autonomy and choice in what we think and what we want because as Harari says, we have become hackable humans.[203] We think we know what we want and what

---

202 Harari, Yuval. 2018. "Why Technology Favors Tyranny." *The Atlantic.* Accessed November 8 2019. https://www.theatlantic.com/magazine/archive/2018/10/yuval-noah-harari-technology-tyranny/568330/.

203 Harari, Yuval N. *21 Lessons for the 21st Century* London: Jonathan Cape, 2018.

we don't want and that we have the option to opt in or out of certain ideas and trends. But really, marketing, social media, and advertising are controlling our wants and needs. In the beauty industry this is extremely relevant. If the consumer is not confident or does not have a good sense of where they stand, what they believe in, and what their style/personality/look represents, it is very easy to get carried away by a false perception of homogenous beauty and we find ourselves striving to reach a certain vision of "perfection."

You're probably thinking: "But, we don't live in a utopia where we can expect all people to intake all of this content positively." True, we don't.

There is another reality, especially in millennials and Generation Zers. It is hardest for us—I include myself because I am in between the two generations, being born in 1996. Technology has slowed the process of our self-exploration because now we are able to live through other people's lives and experiences, let it be our friends or people that we admire, and less of our own tangible experiences. Sometimes even our own experiences we do less for ourselves and more for our followers and friends. The phrases "Do it for the Vine" or "Do it for the Gram" continue to interrupt a peaceful, funny, or engaging moment with friends in order to snap a photo or video.

SWEET, SWEET, PHOTOSHOP

Take a couple of seconds, look at yourself in the mirror and ask yourself: *"Do I feel beautiful?"*

Then look at your social media profiles and ask yourself again: *"Do I feel beautiful?"*

Susana Martinez Vidal[204] shared her thoughts on re-touching photographs.

> I remember a cover that we made in 2009 for *Spanish Elle Magazine* "12 Mujeres (Sobrenaturales)," in English, "12 (Supernatural) Women." These women looked as if they had just woken up. No foundation, no powder, no blush, no nothing. The Spanish models who participated were Elsa Pataky, Sara Carbonero, Paz Vega, and Patricia Conde. They put themselves at the front of *Elle's* cover "Without makeup, without touch-ups, and without fear," as the models claimed. This was primarily done to see

204 Susana Martinez Vidal is a journalist and author, founder of *Ragazza* magazine, which catapulted her to becoming the youngest director of any edition of *Elle* in the world. After seeing the first exhibit of Frida Kahlo's clothing at the Casa Azul in 2012, she was inspired to write her first book, *Frida Kahlo: Fashion as the Art of Being*, recommended by *The New York Times* and *Vanity Fair* UK—most important magazines in more than twenty countries.

the sociological reaction this cover would receive. It was a cover with no photoshop.

I think the photoshop is dangerous if used in the wrong way. Imagine, if we are photoshopping models who are already physically quasi-perfect, it is irrational to want to compare yourself to that. Because of this, the general public has fostered a lot of insecurities and caused a hostile distance between them and icons of beauty.

Influencers, on the other hand, have come closer to society than any admired person before. A lot of them portray their lives in a much more real way. People have more interest in following someone they can more easily aspire to become someday. Just imagine, back in my day magazines were the beauty bible. Models and actresses set the standard, and let me tell you, it was a very narrow standard to follow. Now even influencers are on the covers of Magazines. The demand to normalize beauty icons is evident.

THEY SAY, WE DO

There is something to be said about the way we consume advertisements nowadays. Both Generation Zers and millennials are so attached to the silver screens, especially through Instagram with a culture of living vicariously through our friends or people we admire—call them influencers, KOLs, actresses, models, celebrities, your brother's friend's girlfriend, you name it. I am no psychologist, but I have noticed an interesting phenomenon happening amongst the people around me. It is the way our generations engage with digital and social media beauty advertisements and how this affects our purchasing behaviors.

We are on our phones for hours a day scrolling on Instagram through people's photographs and in the midst of it all pop-up some "serendipitous" sponsors. These are different than ads we were used to seeing before on Facebook, news sites, or other platforms. We are now consuming promotions in the same form as we are consuming content of our friends on vacation, our favorite recipes, or our favorite influencer's outfit for the day. Our brain doesn't differentiate the sponsors from content we choose to consume in our down time that usually takes us to a comfort zone. When we see this on a fast scroll, as they almost look the same, we hold a subconscious feeling of comfort toward the sponsored item or idea.

Talking to Hannah Cecille about this idea,[205] she agreed that our subconscious could be equating these ads to pictures of

---

205 Hannah Cecille is currently a Creative Producer for the largest account on the platform (@Instagram). She is an empathetic storyteller and host who believes it is her purpose to share the stories of underrepresented communities in the world.

our friends and people we are fond of, therefore changing the game of advertising as a whole. Just picture scrolling down numerous pictures of your friends and then, BAM! there is a sponsor of a serum you have never seen before. Maybe you are intrigued by the marketing or the aesthetics of the packaging and you click on it to research further. But most of the time, people swipe down to the next image without giving too much importance to the sponsor.

The idea remains that your subconscious is giving it the same importance as it is giving the picture of your friend and therefore it stays in your memory. Then, when you go to Sephora, Bluemercury, Walmart, CVS, or other, there are so many options for you to choose from. However, you immediately gravitate toward the product that was sponsored on your feed one day and registered in your brain as "trustworthy." This occurs because of the way you consumed the sponsored content when it was introduced to you for the first time. Honestly, this is quite genius on Instagram's part. We as consumers need to be conscious and not allow ourselves to be passive and therefore be hackable humans.

Dr. Sturm[206] says:

---

206 Dr. Barbara Sturm is the founder and CEO of Dr. Barbara Sturm Molecular Cosmetics. She is a German aesthetics doctor, widely renowned for her anti-inflammatory philosophy and her non-surgical anti-aging skin treatments. Dr. Sturm translated science from her clinical research and orthopedic practice into the field of aesthetics and has been a success ever since.

In my opinion technology can make us see something that is different and that is more authentic. We are all so accustomed to seeing perfect women, that it takes a very confident woman like myself, or Gwyneth Paltrow[207] to appear just as we are, to make people realize beauty can be natural. Because in the end you decide how you look on social media. You decide if you put a filter on a picture or spend time editing the picture to look like something else.

I have witnessed this phenomenon with myself and speaking to many of my beauty-obsessed friends. We find ourselves buying certain products for an odd "unexplainable" reason that seems to be glanced over. It is merely impossible to think this will subside or can be changed, but, on the contrary, I think this emotional subconscious connection will be the future of successful marketing. The only thing we can currently do is be more aware because awareness is intelligence. When you see a product that looks appealing, research it further and have a conscious look for a minute to register it as a sponsor.

---

207 Gweneth Paltrow is an American actress, singer, author, and beauty guru, and businesswoman, CEO, and founder of Goop, a natural health, beauty, and lifestyle brand.

TOO MUCH TRUST

We trust influencers, KOLs and celebrities to have done their due diligence when speaking about the products they are promoting, and we rely on their judgment to purchase it or not. I, myself, am guilty of this. However, I always try to do my own research on the side to assure myself that what I am buying is of quality.

The danger is that we feel confident about our own judgement after learning from influencers, even if what they are saying is not entirely true. However, since they explain information in a more digestible manner for the busy consumer, they are able to sway us one way or the other about a product. This of course happens in every dimension of the consumerist world, but for the beauty industry, it is especially relevant. Because brands have a lot less power on what they say about their products, the consumer and influencers have more power than ever to promote these or not on social media.

In *21st Lessons for the 21st Century*,[208] Harari, turns his attention to the present. He attempts to untangle the technological, political, social, and existential predicaments that humankind faces. Harari says there is something to

---

208 *21st Lessons for the 21st Century* is a book written by bestseller Israeli author Yuval Noah Harari and published in August 2018 preceding the books *Sapiens: A Brief History of HumanKind* (2011) and *Homo Deus: A Brief History of Tomorrow* (2016)

be said about the model in which we consume news and information. [209] We have constructed a model that follows the rule of receiving news for free in exchange for human attention. More and more competition for exciting news is going on at the moment. However, the quality of that news is questionable.

We seem to be triggered by news that sparks an emotion, instead of news that correctly informs us. Some of the most intelligent people in the world have learned how to make news appealing enough for us to click on their resources instead of others', and in turn the quality information gets pushed aside. What is interesting is that people are willing to pay for high-quality food, cars, education, and clothes, yet many are still not willing to pay for high-quality news. [210]

The beauty industry is becoming more and more saturated with information—true information and false information—but it is hard to tell them apart. This causes a problem because it is easy to be lured in the wrong direction out of pure confusion. Yet, there is a bright side. We have the luxury to have a saturated market because if we are educated about what we want and what we need, we can find a brand that caters to us exactly. The more the beauty industry becomes

209 Harari, Yuval N. 21 Lessons for the 21st Century London: Jonathan Cape, 2018.
210 Ibid.

inclusive, the more space in the market will open for niche brands to fill.

We have to be careful though, Yuval Noah Harari also suggests in *21st Lessons for the 21st Century,* that our ability to manipulate ourselves is increasing, especially for millennials and Generation Zers. We need to make sure we have a better understanding of our identity in order to be more compassionate toward ourselves. [211] Harari claims that our society has been advancing at such tremendous speeds with social media, technology, and even the advent of AI and VR, that we are having to adapt to an excessively stimulating world. [212] We are now losing our own choices to commercialism, advertising, and marketing more than ever before, and these generations are the most affected.[213]

At this pace, there is no way we can predict the future of beauty, but emerging brands and indie brands have a chance to steer and help consumers adapt their perception of beauty toward a more representative one.

The only way to beat the stimulation is knowing ourselves better.

---

211 Ibid.
212 Ibid.
213 Ibid.

There is no point in deleting Snapchat, Facebook, or Instagram because all of those are platforms are almost a necessity in today's norm to be in the know of what is going on. But we need to improve our emotional intelligence, understand who we are, and cultivate our inner beauty.

You must learn to celebrate your uniqueness instead of waiting on someone else to do so on your behalf.

THE COMFORT SYNDROME

The dark side of technology rises as we lose our own sense of self. The plastic surgery and noninvasive cosmetic treatment industry is making lots of people lose their compass. The increased comparison technology prompts us to do also allows people all over the world to discover certain trends in features that are "in," such a lip fillers, for example. Feature trends don't have to be bad unless you are subscribing to them to look like everyone else, and not to make yourself *feel* more beautiful and content with yourself.

As consumers we must stay aware of the negative aspects of falling into copycat trends. For example, have you ever heard women say, "When I was younger the trendiest eyebrows were the ones that were pencil thin. Now, I can't grow mine out any longer!" I bet you have. Back then many women subscribed that trend, and as a result, now they are finding it hard to subscribe to the thicker eyebrow trend.

What if we all wore the eyebrow shape and thickness we thought went best with the rest of our face?

I think it would be a lot more original, interesting, and beautiful.

It's unfortunate that the beauty industry is serving as a tool to not enhance, but rather, completely change one's features to look like a 180K follower-backed influencer from SoHo. We have headed into some murky waters of technology and homogeneous beauty.

Nayera Senane[214] sees this in her practice as Botox and dermal filler lip injector. She says that most millennials who get their lips done with her "pop a picture from an influencer on Instagram" to show what they want their lips to resemble. "It's a millennial thing," she says. I think depending on the intention the person has when showing this picture, this isn't always a toxic practice. It can help the doctor to know what the patient's goal is to better meet the patient's needs.

---

214 Nayera Senane is a Diamond Allergan Injector, Botox and dermal filler expert. She currently holds a wide client base including celebrities and models. Although based in Los Angeles, she travels regularly to the East Coast to see clients.

But overall, comparison brings patients to lose their sense of what would look good on them versus what looks good on someone else. Ultimately, I believe you should trust your doctor to enhance your look to fit you and not change what inherently is *you*—of course, only if it is a well-known experienced doctor.

Influencers, actresses, models, and celebrities, being more comfortable with posting about their facial alterations and enhancements, have certainly made something that was taboo, like facial modifications, a mainstream. As Nayera mentions:

> Before people were more private about cosmetic surgery and wanted to keep it as natural as possible. Kylie Jenner really pioneered the less natural look into a standard of beauty, especially when speaking about lips. I have noticed that in the last five years women have been more confident asking for bigger lips. They don't mind being swollen later either. Many of them post about the results right after I finish with them on their social media and others even document it while it's happening.

Although it may seem like it with all this talk, I am by no means opposed to cosmetic alterations and enhancements. I believe if you want to enhance yourself to highlight your own look, identity, or features—go for it! However, I am not a big fan of changing your features to look like someone else. Instead of using social media to contemplate how to conform to the looks of another person, I encourage you to use it as a tool to *feel* more beautiful. You may think, well social media only makes you feel less beautiful because there are so many incredible stunning girls on social media. But really, it is all about how you look at this tool. By appreciating all the different beauties out there in the world and having the opportunity to see these beauties, you have that 360 view at your fingertips. Hopefully you see that beauty does not look one way or another by seeing this array of images of beauty on social media.

Jeanne Chavez gracefully phrased her point of view on the trend that technology is prompting.

There's always the overly exaggerated and the really understated. They always live in the same place, and people usually get labeled one or the other.

What I think is so fantastic is social media has allowed us to have an almost bird's eye view into all these different trends—what you like, or what you align with, or what makes you feel like you. We didn't have that before. We just had TV, movies, or fashion magazines to look at what beauty was which was, so limited compared to what we have now.

I'm not here to judge any of it. But I do think overly exaggerated features are always going to be around no matter what times we live in. Yet, the same way we have the "fake look" trend, we have the all-natural trend. Both extremes will always live together.

I mean, to me, it is a luxury to have this choice. I really enjoy the freedom that people have to make those choices. They live together beautifully. They always have.

As Jeanne says, it is a question of accepting that it's a revolutionary concept to have so much choice about what your perception of beauty is and how you will apply it to yourself. Social media has gifted us with this choice.

It is all about digesting the panoramic view of beauty we have so easily accessible to us and taking in what is necessary to make you feel beautiful, not your followers. Your perception of beauty is a choice and not a standard.

EMOTIONALLY ATTACHED TO DIGITAL CONTENT

Consumers in general are beginning to feel a deeper emotional attachment to brands. A great example of this is SKII with their PITERA Essence video content describing the "legend" of this product through a comical video series of #PITERAmasterclass featuring celebrities from all over the world: James Corden (English), Naomi Watanabe (Japanese), Tang Wei (Chinese), and John Legend (American). With this content, formulation SKII did an outstanding job of making the product known to different communities through a form of digestible information. One of my favorites is the "Oh, Pitera" song by John Legend explaining what PITERA does to your skin.

Consumers feel an emotional connection to the SKII brand and its products for many different reasons: celebrities, inclusive representation of race, gender, and culture, and even just the effectiveness of this ancient formula. They feel like this makes the brand immediately more relatable regardless whether you know the exact ingredients, formulation, safety, or potency—which for SKII, happen to be excellent. I am a PITERA Essence fan myself.

Another example of effective consumer engagement is through the representative influencers who promote a brand itself. Jacinda Heintz,[215] one of Ole Henriksen's brand influencers, pushes for an aspect of beauty that transcends all cultural nuances: self-confidence, self-love, and personal health. Through her posts, a brand can demonstrate the products and their uses through content on Instagram and IGTV (Instagram TV). This type of content creates a more interactive experience for social audiences and cuts through the typical social marketing noise.

> I think influencer marketing creates more validity for brands with consumers by having products endorsed by these public figures that audiences build a level of trust with. However, consumers are smarter than ever and can easily cut through the noise of a paid partnership that is not organic. Social audiences pay attention to these details and in order for a partnership to seem seamless, it's important that both the influencer and brand are a fit for one another.
>
> —JACINDA HEINTZ

According to an article on *Business Insider*, it is projected that the influencer market will be a ten-billion-dollar industry

---

215 Jacinda Heintz is an Influencer Marketing Coordinator at Kendo Brands, Inc. She leverages her social media and marketing expertise to create socially driven partnerships that are mutually beneficial for both the brand and the influencer.

by 2020.[216] This rapid growth in such a young industry is one we must pay attention to. Instagram influencer partnerships receive an average of 3.21 percent engagement rate from consumers compared to a 1.5 percent across other social media platforms—making Instagram the highest performing platform for brands to invest their marketing budgets to see maximum exposure.[217]

Influencer Marketing is becoming one of the most lucrative mediums to market, if it is done honestly and genuinely. According to Linqia's reports survey, *The State of Influencer Marketing Survey*, where 197 marketers participated, it was revealed that 39 percent of marketers plan to increase their influencer marketing budget in 2019. This decision was based on the data that 68 percent of marketers cite Instagram as the most important social network.[218] Fifty-seven percent of companies and brands reported that influencer content outperformed brand-created content, leaving it clear this is the path

---

216 "INFLUENCER MARKETING 2019: Why Brands Can'T Get Enough Of An $8 Billion Ecosystem Driven By Kardashians, Moms, And Tweens." 2019. Business Insider France. Accessed November 5 2019. https://www.businessinsider.fr/us/ the-2019-influencer-marketing-report-2019-7.

217 "This Is How Much Instagram Influencers Really Cost." 2019. *Later Blog.* Accessed October 2 2019. https://later.com/blog/ instagram-influencers-costs/.

218 2019. *Linqia.Com.* Accessed October 2 2019. https://linqia. com/wp-content/uploads/2019/04/Linqia-State-of-Influencer-Marketing-2019-Report.pdf.

to take in terms of marketing.[219] In fact, it is so evident that Estée Lauder's CEO, Fabrizio Freda, revealed in August 2019, that this multinational beauty company will now be spending 75 percent of its marketing budget on influencers.[220]

Due to this generation's craving to feel included and cared about, the influencer marketing is skyrocketing. When consumers view influencer-created content and it seems genuine, they relate to it and feel comfortable. We believe the influencer has done their homework, and they know better than us what we should be buying and using.

Harvard Business School article, "Lipstick Tips: How Influencers Are Making Over Beauty Marketing," supports that influencer marketing has become one of the most effective ways to reach beauty consumers, creating cult-like followings—notably on YouTube with Vloggers and Instagram with influencers.[221] These have become the most trustworthy ways to pitch products according to Alessia Vettese's research, a Harvard Business School MBA graduate student.

219 Ibid.
220 Pearl, Diana, and Diana Pearl. 2019. "75 percent Of Estée Lauder's Marketing Budget Is Going To Digital—And Influencers." *Adweek. Com.* Accessed October 2 2019. https://www.adweek.com/brand-marketing/75-of-estee-lauders-marketing-budget-is-going-to-influencers/.
221 Ibid.

People used to watch celebrities on the red carpet talking about what they were wearing, or they would flip through magazines and look at celebrities in makeup ads, but that has lost its traction, especially among younger consumers. Now, people want to go online and get an at-your-fingertips experience. They want to ask an influencer questions and get personal responses.

—ALESSIA VETTESE.[222]

Vettese surveyed 520 women, targeting beauty enthusiasts on social media, and she found the following results to her question: "Where do you seek information about beauty products before you buy?"[223]

Social Media Influencers:	67 percent
Third-Party Reviews:	59 percent
Beauty Professionals:	55 percent
Professional Networks:	48 percent
Company Advertisements:	44 percent
Public Figures/Celebrities:	34 percent

222 Ibid.
223 Ibid.

This survey proves that the generations of today are devoted to following the lives of people who have similar lifestyles to them or who resonate with them in some way or another, being the highest solicited channel for product information.

I believe one reason amongst many is that influencers we follow are "experiencing" products on our behalf, which in a way could be replacing the "free trial" period we are so attached to. Since they have "tried" it, we feel more comfortable buying the products without asking additional questions.

WE THINK INFLUENCERS ARE OUR BEST FRIENDS

According to IZEA,[224] some of the most popular beauty influencers at for 2019 are:

- Rihanna
- Kylie Jenner
- Naomi Giannopoulos
- Zoe Sugg
- Kandee Johnson
- Genelle Seldon
- Jeffree Star
- Tati Westbrook

---

224 "The Top Beauty and Makeup Artist Influencers of 2019." 2019. *IZEA*. Accessed October 2 2019. https://izea.com/2019/02/01/makeup-artist/.

- James Charles
- Jaclyn Hill
- Laura Lee
- Desi Perkins
- Huda Kattan
- Nikkie de Jager
- Manny Mua
- Aaron Storms

If you are a makeup buff, you may religiously follow some of these people and you might feel they have opened up to you so much that you know them on a deeper level.

In Vettese's study, she found that one of the reasons why one can become emotionally attached to influencers is because they do not just talk about beauty products. They expose their life in such an intimate way—showing video and visual content of their family, friends, trips, pets, kids, alone-time, insecurities, places they frequent, their travel, their cooking, and lifestyle routines. [225] Sometimes, we can know more about James Charles than we would know our own friends.

---

225 Pearl, Diana, and Diana Pearl. 2019. "75 percent Of Estée Lauder's Marketing Budget Is Going To Digital—And Influencers." Adweek.Com. Accessed October 2 2019. https://www.adweek. com/brand-marketing/75-of-estee-lauders-marketing-budget-is-going-to-influencers/.

Vettese says: "These consumers are building relationships, and they are bonding with these influencers. They have regular conversations back and forth, and they think of the influencers as being directly ingrained in their day-to-day lives." [226]

But Don't Be Fooled...

No matter where one stands socio-economically, everyone is willing to save and invest in looking their best. For this reason, the last thing a consumer would want is for a product to reverse the "beautifying effect" we so hoped to get. Which could be the case, if we buy a product that is not meant for us.

Three years ago, one of my favorite micro-influencers spoke about a magic chemical peel she had done and how amazing it had left her face. Me, as a beauty enthusiast who was not yet knowledgeable or conscious about the way I consumed beauty, went ahead and booked an appointment to get this peel done. My skin was healthy, and nothing was really wrong with it at all except from some breakouts here and there. Do not try to fix what is not broken. Perfection is not beauty.

This treatment was a significant investment and it completely backfired on my skin. I was flacking for a few weeks, which

---

226 Ibid.

is normal, but then I began to have rough patches in certain parts of my face. It took my skin about six months to recover with the help of Maria Calderon's[227] formulations and knowledge. This is a perfect example of why you should not be a passive beauty consumer and not do all you are told on social media by your influencer "best friends" or sponsors.

Do your research, be conscious, and pay attention to things you want to invest in. Make sure they do not reverse your "beauty-fully" healthy skin and make sure what you are investing in is right for you.

When we feel that our "best friend" influencer has tried it, and they claim they love it, we are more likely to believe the product or treatment must work. Suddenly, all the fear of buying an expensive beauty product that might not be effective is removed. The amount of trust that we put in these influencers is dangerous because a lot of times the products they are promoting are not products they truly believe in. Rather, they are paid to showcase them. Influencers can get paid astronomical amounts to post one piece of content with a product or brand or even just mention one in a post.

---

227 Maria Calderon is the CEO and founder of Kosmetai, founder of Institut Nahia, and founder of Juveskin, S.L. company, where she serves as Director General and is the Technical Director of PRODUCTOS BIORGANICOS, S.L. Maria is a chemical cosmetic pharmaceutical specialist and licensed expert in the evaluation of the security and information files of cosmetic products.

The good news is that we are quickly becoming aware of the fact that this is a problem and more and more consumers are beginning to be skeptical of what celebrities models, and influencers promote. This is a good thing because although they do believe in what they post at times, it is a great habit to do your own research on the side. Vettese finds more credibility in the influencers who give some products good reviews and others more negative ones. It also helps when the influencer, model or celeb, outwardly claims that they are not being sponsored by any brand—making them more legitimate sources.

One consumer in Vettese's study said:

> Kim Kardashian promotes all kinds of products all the time that I'm skeptical she uses. She'll post an Instagram holding a jar of Olay, for example, but then you'll read an interview where she says she always uses a $1,000 Guerlain cream. A celebrity putting their name on something isn't really enough to draw me in by itself. [228]

---

228 Pearl, Diana, and Diana Pearl. 2019. "75 percent Of Estée Lauder's Marketing Budget Is Going To Digital—And Influencers." *Adweek. Com.* Accessed October 2 2019. https://www.adweek.com/brand-marketing/75-of-estee-lauders-marketing-budget-is-going-to-influencers/.

It is clear that we are becoming subjects to influencer marketing, which again has two sides to it. It could be the most legitimate form of marketing if we know how to choose our influencers correctly and conduct fact checking ourselves, or it could be a complete case of "they say, we do." That is what makes us hackable humans.

The saddening part for me is that most of us think we are making an educated decision because we trust what we read and consume on digital media too much.

Stay cautious. Stay aware and be a smart consumer.

We are what we consume, not only orally, but visually as well.

PART III

HOW WE SUCCEED

CHAPTER 7

HONOR YOURSELF

———

With the copious amounts of visual content available to us at a moment's notice, we spend the vast majority of our time looking at our own faces or those of others. As a result, either implicitly or explicitly, we are constantly learning what beauty "should" look like.

We often focus so much on what beauty looks like that we forget what beauty *feels* like. This is how one exudes their beauty and how one radiates energy, which in my opinion is the most central component of beauty.

A perception of beauty that celebrates unique features has the power to make our society live more confidently. *Feeling* beautiful is a right that every human being has. It is one that should be endorsed more by society so each and every one of us can feel like the best versions of ourselves every day of our lives. People will be empowered to feel more confident in all aspects of life.

DIGITAL LIFE: DOWN A RABBIT HOLE

Huge steps backward are taken when people prioritize *looks* rather than *feels*.

There is a deep, dark and terrifying side of social media that we have not quite yet touched on—the forum sphere of beauty. This world is fueled by objective, measurable, visible, obsessive, hateful, and completely toxic definitions of beauty. These definitions come from the feeling of needing to subscribe to society's standard image of beauty—quite literally one found by analyzing the geometry of the top most attractive models and celebrities deemed by society.

I had the opportunity to speak with a young woman[229] who suffered a lot in her experience through hateful beauty forums. To this day, she is haunted by flashbacks and intermittent insecurity that she hopes one day will leave her memory. While hearing her story I was completely taken aback by the extent to which beauty forums can destroy one's inner beauty.

---

229 This person wishes to keep personal information anonymous.

This young woman was brave and opened up to me about her story. She told me the following:

> When I started university and looked around at all the beautiful girls who walked around campus, I felt incredibly self-conscious about my appearance. I compared myself to all of them. They were just so beautiful! After all, I was at one of the most notorious universities for "hot girls."
>
> I was suddenly very aware of everything "wrong" with my face. New insecurities popped up every day:
>
> Was my nose too wide?
>
> Were my lips too narrow?
>
> Was my face too chubby?
>
> In search of the truth about how I really looked, I started going online to beauty forums. I surfed them quite often and then decided to start posting my pictures in rating forums myself.
>
> The idea was simple: post a few photos of yourself from different angles and let people tell you how

beautiful you are, as well as the flaws that hold you back.

The first few times I posted the comments were flattering... a little too good to be true for my insecure-self who saw myself as average at the very best. I went deeper into the web, posting to increasingly more obscure websites, and getting sucked into the darker side of the beauty debate.

That's where I stumbled upon "incels," which is short for "involuntarily celibate" men who blame women for their lack of sexual activity and essentially, their misery in life. Mostly, they wallowed in their own physical insecurities and criticize women, targeting their supposed shallowness and how they always date stereotypically attractive popular males instead of being interested in them. Basically, incels believe that if women were more attractive, they would have better luck in sex, love, and life—never mind their personal characteristics and inner-beauty. This mindset led to dozens of these men posting ratings on pictures of women's faces on such forums, giving comments about what prevents them from being attractive. But it was never a simple case of, "you're too short" or "your eyebrows are too bushy." Incels have boiled down beauty and beauty standards to a science. They analyze each face down to the most minor of details.

But what made these websites especially toxic, among other things, is the behavior they displayed toward women who posted there—including me.

I remember the first time I posted there. I had a thought, "They couldn't possibly find THAT many things wrong with my face." I was self-conscious but not to an extreme level. Well, not yet at least.

All it took was the first few comments to completely destroy my self-esteem. I became insecure about body parts I didn't even know existed, and things I didn't even know I had to be insecure about, like the softness of my facial features, the height of my cheekbones, and the position of my lips relative to my nose. I was completely decimated. I ended up deleting that first post and obsessing about my features for the next few weeks, trying to improve each flaw they had pointed out in the forum with facial exercises, makeup, and weight loss. A month later, I came back to the group with more photos, hoping my reviews would improve. They did, but only incrementally. None contained the validation I was hoping for. This led to a cycle of me posting on the websites over and over again. Each time, the feedback was so different that the backlash of the varying comments only increased my insecurity. I became nearly underweight hoping to satisfy their standards, to the point where even the commenters pointed out how skinny I had become. But the ratings kept going up, so I kept posting for that new dose of validation every time. I just wanted to *feel* beautiful.

What made me finally stop and realize how toxic these websites are was looking at the comments on other girls' posts and realizing how ridiculous they were. These incel raters, who were mostly male, were picking apart beautiful young women's faces that had nothing wrong with them. Moreover, their comments were combined with clearly racist and sexist undertones. That's what destroyed their credibility in my eyes. Slowly, I started my ascent out of the hellhole I had fallen into.

Even though I stopped going and posting on the forums, I still struggled to get rid of that toxically detailed view of beauty I had fallen into. What made this struggle so difficult was looking at ads and magazines around me. No matter how much I told myself that every single aspect of their aesthetic theories were ridiculous and that everyone's beauty was unique, I couldn't help but notice that the women who were chosen to model adhered pretty closely to the standards on those online forums. Almost all of them had similar features of almond-shaped eyes, sharp high cheekbones, and thin noses, making me struggle with the concept that my own face was beautiful.

Years later, I can finally say I've learned to look at myself in the mirror and not dissect my face into parts and problems anymore. But, that's not to say that my experiences haven't left an impact on my self-image. Every now and then I can slip up and find myself drawn to beauty products that mention "fillers" or "filler-like effect" on the box, implying they could permanently change my face for the better.

Over time, these habits have been slowly disappearing as I've changed my perception of beauty. I noticed that every time I went out feeling confident and in a good mood, people would be more drawn to me than if I had contoured my nose differently that morning; paradoxically, people's external perception of me depended on my internal beauty.

Now, instead of trying to adhere to the ever-changing standards on online forums or even those in the beauty industry, I try to be the best version of myself and highlight what I'm happy with and proud of, and eventually learn to love the rest.

I am now more interested in exercising and using cruelty-free makeup with natural ingredients that would enhance my features instead of changing them. Even though it has been a long and hard battle to get to the place I am now, my deeper sense of satisfaction with myself and how I look has been endlessly worth it.

I highly advise you not to ever indulge in any of these forums, and if you find yourself doing so, please seek help. I really cannot stress enough how important it is not only to cultivate our beauty from within and make sure we have the strength, confidence, and mindset to *feel* powerful and confident. Validation of your beauty and self-worth has to come from yourself, rather than from others or even online strangers.

These are the dangers of viewing beauty objectively and as something purely physical. Unfortunately, numerous young women share experiences such as the one above. There are real dangers that we need to protect each other from, and we can do so by understanding beauty in a more holistic manner. Many people who are posting on these websites are Gen Zers, millennials, and even some Generation Xers. These toxic rating forums have often come close to being banned due to the severe effects they have on young women, and even some men. However, they have found their way to remain online.

Cara Delevingne, a British model and actress, posted on her Instagram on September 5, 2019, a picture of a quote saying: "When you admire something about another woman, tell her. Get into the habit of lifting each other up."

—UNKNOWN

Social media is no longer used merely to socialize, but also to spread messages and images of good and unfortunately also of evil, causing a backlash and triggering mental health issues, depression, and even suicide. This is especially true with user generated content platforms.

The key is to know where and when to stop yourself from going into a rabbit hole and the dark world of the web. It can be complicated at times to find a level of moderation, since our lives now seem to revolve around social media and the internet. Nowadays, we have a question and we google it.

Beauty exists in everyone, and it only takes one person to point out someone's unique beauty for that individual to be uplifted.

WORK LIFE: AS WOMEN IN THE WORKFORCE

We all want to *feel* represented and understood. This goes for women who are working mothers, and consequently, have little time for themselves, as well. The want to see beauty accessible to them as they do not have much time themselves to spend on their beauty. But as every woman, they still want to *feel* beautiful.

These women face a lot of pressure. Not only are they required by society to have an incredible career, look beautiful, have kids, and cook, but we are also expected to do all of this without limits! Although this can be a conversation of fairness or not, if anyone can do it, women can.

We, as women, have the privilege—at least in my opinion—of being able to adorn and pamper ourselves to *feel* the best possible version of ourselves. When we are not in a good state of mind, we can do a little pampering and alter our mood for the better at least a little.

Personally, I put on some sweet-smelling perfume, lip-gloss and, a little mascara, *et voila* a completely renewed me. For others, it is red lipstick or a little bit of blush. Whatever you want to do, you can do it to *feel* like you will *seize the day* and be that heroine for yourself. We need to be able to express ourselves in a way that makes us *feel* like we can perform best in our personal lives and be efficient, confident, and successful in our day-to-day. The good thing is that as women we have so many opportunities to do so!

In some industries, there are strong incentives for women to pamper themselves before work and look "presentable" for the workplace, yet, in others it is almost frowned upon. Some women find it a relief that they don't need to worry about looking nice for work, but others would love to be able to express themselves and wear a little something to *feel* their best self.

Of course, makeup and skin care are not the answer to all problems, but if they can help us *feel* better, why not use them to our advantage? A report on the state of self-esteem by the Dove Self-Esteem Fund (2008) stated that "78 percent of girls with low self-esteem admit that it's hard to feel good in school when you don't feel good about how you look (compared to 54 percent of girls with high self-esteem)."[230]

When you *feel* good about yourself you walk a different way.

Jeanne Chavez says:

230 "Why More Women Are Happily Going Without Makeup." 2019. Psychology Today. Accessed October 2 2019. https://www.psychologytoday.com/ca/blog/the-clarity/201707/why-more-women-are-happily-going-without-makeup.

If you put even the slightest little bit of makeup or skin care on, you do your hair, you do basic hygiene, or simply show that you gave yourself at least ten minutes of priority before stepping out into the world, people react to you differently. Why? Because that shows a level of respect and self-love you have for yourself and people absolutely pick up on that.

What usually happens is that if you walk out of the house looking messy, it can be inferred by others that you *feel* that way inside too.

It's like the famous line, "Dress for Success," but with beautifying self-care.

When you walk out of your house, and you *feel* like you've really put some time and effort into your hygiene, skin, makeup, hair—your "vehicle" as I like to call it—people tend to react differently toward you.

Jeanne says:

People treat you with a little bit more courtesy and respect because they're honoring what you've just put into your look for the day. It might sound superficial, but honestly my whole career has been built on that and I really believe in it. It works for me, it works for my children, it works for my husband. It is not just for women. It's for all genders too...It really is just about the effort someone puts into taking care of themselves and the way they carry themselves. Your appearance is the transmitter of the immeasurable beauty inside of you.

WORK LIFE: A HINDU WOMAN IN STEM

Some women in STEM jobs want to be beautiful and empowered but, many women in these fields have felt there is no space for beauty in the office. A lot of them wish they could feel feminine and put together but *feel* as if work is not the place to do it.

You spend most of the hours of your week in the office at work, though, so where do it if not there?

In our conversation about cultures and their different approaches to beauty in the workforce, Meghna Chakraborty[231] shared an interesting story about her mother.

---

231 Meghna Chakraborty is now a graduate student at the University of Southern California. Previously, she was a content strategy intern at Live Tinted, a multicultural beauty brand. Driven by her passion for innovative experiences and diverse storytelling, she is determined to help elevate unheard voices and underrepresented faces in media and pop culture.

It is a great way to highlight the restrictions that women in STEM fields feel in this regard.

Meghna's mother works in Silicon Valley, and all throughout Meghna's childhood she never saw her mother wearing much makeup at all. She would only wear a certain type of eye liner from India, Kajal and sometimes red lipstick, but never to work. Meghna explained that this was only propagated due to the field her mother was in. She says, "In STEM jobs, it is already rare to find women. It is even rarer to find women who are encouraged to look the best versions of themselves." In my opinion there needs to be a more open and inclusive environment in the workforce, no matter what field you are in, that allows you to be you as you wish, without feeling pressure to look one way or another.

Meghna's mother believes that *feeling* beautiful at work is reserved for people in other fields, and that shouldn't be the case. In Meghna's perspective, this is not just a problem as a result of the women or men in STEM. It is because the branding of beauty brands is not catering to this market. In other words, brands are not granting these women the possibility to *feel* beautiful because there are no examples of women in stem behind beauty marketing, billboards, and brands. But, influencers of all levels are beginning to show a more empowering image of women, representing in fact women in stem who look exactly as they would like at work.

Beauty brands should make a more concentrated effort to represent women in the workforce. Everyone has a right to *feel* beautiful. It does not make sense to have to choose between *feeling* beautiful and a successful career.

WORK LIFE: BLACK WOMAN RADIATING BEAUTY ON WALL STREET

Understanding what success looks like as well as understanding yourself and your unique talents is what lets your inner beauty shine through. No one will question your ability to succeed if you *feel* confident, appear assured of your capabilities, and consistently foster your potential.

Passion, determination, and energy to do something for yourself and for others.

I like to call these intangibles. They are *je ne sais quoi* that brings out that charismatic presence.

One incredible example of a woman who embodies her beauty on Wall Street is Chinwe Esimai.[232] Chinwe is one

---

232 Chinwe Esimai is the Managing Director and Chief Anti-Bribery Officer at Citigroup, Inc. She is also an award-winning lawyer, author, and speaker who is passionate about inspiring generations of immigrant women leaders.

of the most beautiful women I have ever met; you don't need to look at her for longer than three seconds to know this woman *feels* beautiful too. She carries herself with such a firm identity and confidence that she makes you want to talk to her all day long.

In our conversation, Chinwe recalled a story that reassured me of how far you can get in life when you know your self-worth.

> I think what makes me radiate is confidence. This confidence stems from knowledge and experience, beginning with the knowledge I gained in college and law school, but perhaps more importantly, it stems from a sense of knowing my purpose. Early on, I knew I wanted to work in something that impacted not just the US, but also Nigeria, the developing world, and indeed, the rest of the world. Considering that I moved to the United States from Nigeria in my teens, I had developed a global view and a passion to impact the world.
>
> I started my professional career at a law firm and subsequently worked at Goldman Sachs. At some point, I realized I was interested in anti-bribery work because I believed I could add value in this field. When I finally got the opportunity to work in

this area, I realized I really enjoyed it. Eventually, this blossomed into my present role at Citibank.

I've always been a hard worker. I approach my work with excellence and give 110 percent—always. It gives me a sense of accomplishment to bring the best version of myself to work. When I first took on the global role, covering over 160 countries around the world, it was intimidating. There were times I thought I wasn't ready for it, but over time, I gained confidence. I also brought a lot of passion to the role. The seeds of my passion were sewn at a very early age, growing up in a developing country and having a desire to help create ethical business cultures around the world.

The more decisions you make, the more confidence you gain in your decision-making abilities. You also become more confident to advocate for your opinions.

So, what does this have to do with my beauty? I could not have made it this far without believing in myself and in my unique value.

I am grateful for a conversation with a friend of a mentor who gave me very simple advice: "Don't spend your time wondering what others think of your age or what you look like. Doing so will be an enormous distraction to your success."

For me, it is critical to tune in throughout the day through prayer and meditation—in the morning, in the afternoon, and before I go to bed. I am also intentional about my weekly and daily schedules. I set weekly goals, not just for work, but also personal goals for my husband, each of my three kids, and for every single area of my life, ranging from spiritual to financial. I review these goals daily and this helps me continually make progress toward my most important intentions.

Chinwe also noted the importance of living with intention. She says, "Failing to live with intention is a disservice to one's self and to those around you. We must resist the mentality of being busy and distracted because this robs the world of our authentic voice and presence."

WORK LIFE: OWN YOUR HAIR

Chinwe also spoke about her beautiful locks and staying true to how she wants to express her identity through her hair. She says, "The truth is that I have never experienced a negative commentary or discrimination because of my locks at work, neither today, nor years ago when I had short, natural hair."

She noted that the only few negative reactions she received earlier in her career regarding natural hair came from fellow women of color, which is unfortunate, Chinwe believes. She recalled a particular experience when she interviewed with a Caucasian man for a position on Wall Street. She said the interview went fabulous, but his admin (who was also of color), gave her a dirty look as she left the interview, one that seemed to say, *"Where is she going with that hair."* [233]

Chinwe emphasized how significant it is to support, appreciate, and to allow one another to *feel* beautiful in our various expressions of culture and the very expressions that make us *feel* like ourselves.

That goes for anyone really. Support people and allow them to *feel* beautiful.

Say, "THIS is who I AM."

---

233 "Chinwe Esimai, The African Woman Leading Citi's Anti-Bribery & Corruption Efforts." 2019. *Facebook Watch.* Accessed October 3 2019. https://www.facebook.com/Face2FaceAfrica/videos/836609520007529/?v=836609520007529.

Speaking to Kennedy Daniel,[234] an incredible young woman of color who grew up in LA. She is now working part time at Glossier.[235] She explained her transition in the relationship with her own hair before and after her start at this beauty company.

Kennedy grew up with an idea from a young age that in order to be beautiful she had to straighten her hair. This became a habit, and therefore, she never thought twice about it. When she began working at Glossier, where the employees were all incredibly vibrant and diverse, she began to realize the unexpressed potential her hair held and decided to start celebrating it.

Kennedy shares:

> I was the youngest amongst all of the employees and was very impressionable in terms of how appreciative and how encouraging the employees were about me expressing my natural and identity-based beauty.

---

234 Kennedy Daniel works part time at Glossier LA on Melrose Place as an Offline Editor while she finishes her BA at the University of Southern California. Kennedy is proud to say she was a member of the original team of Offline Editors who helped open the store in the Spring of 2018.

235 Glossier is a trendy skin care and makeup brand, providing essentials for dewy, glowing skin from head-to-toe. The brand is valued at $1.2 billion.

I was just eating it all up and felt the most confident I had ever been! This allowed me to see the importance of understanding how to celebrate myself and feel beautiful in my own features and uniqueness. For the first time in as long as I can remember, I started wearing my big curly crazy hair. I let go of the misconception that straight hair was a beauty standard I was supposed to uphold. Being around my colleagues at Glossier makes me feel the most beautiful because they appreciate me and my beauty on a deeper level.

This sentiment of celebrating your unique beauty is felt beyond the employees, but in the store and in each of the products of Glossier. I think this is why we have such loyal consumers. Glossier has products that celebrate you and how you truly look, so often their products are very sheer and light weight, such as the foundation.

At Glossier you really can be creative with products to accentuate your unique features as much as you can. For example, the liquid blush, I put on my eyes, on my lips and on my cheeks. It really makes my melon pop.

A woman said to me one day that she loved putting the Glossier mascara on her eyebrows because she had very thick eyebrows and she wanted to make them even thicker. The pure fact that she did that was so amazing to me because beauty is about how YOU feel and not so much about how a brand tells you a product is supposed to make you feel.

PERSONAL LIFE: SELF-CARE IS "IN," TAKE ADVANTAGE OF IT!

Self-care is a discipline. It is based on the idea of dedicating more time to oneself both physically (masks, treatments, skin cleansing, etc.) and emotionally (holistic therapies, techniques of mindfulness, relaxation, etc.). As a result of the often stressful and overstimulated world we live in, it is now becoming a fad to take care of yourself. What a fantastic trend to follow!

Those of us who experience mental health problems associated with perceptions of beauty often have negative thoughts. Often, those negative thoughts then create unwanted feelings, as Dr. Lauren Hazzouri[236] mentions at BeautyCon LA. After recognizing the feelings, it's equally important to go

---

236 Dr. Lauren Hazzouri is a licensed psychologist, international public speaker, founder of Hazzouri Psychology, Scranton, and founder of NOT THERAPY—a program she created to address the unique mental health concerns of girls and women. She has been named one of the "Top 5 Women in the World Inspiring Girls" by German *Glamour,* and her trailblazing work has appeared in publications including *Teen Vogue, Forbes,* and British *Vogue.*

through your thoughts and analyze which ones are creating unwanted feelings.

To tackle this, Dr. Hazzouri suggests writing down every single negative thought that goes through your head. She says doing this can help you reflect and realize if these thoughts are true or if they are just something you have repeated to yourself enough times that you have convinced yourself they are true.

Because remember, thoughts are thoughts and not facts.

Once you have this, Dr. Hazzouri says you can say to yourself: *"Excuse me, inner critic. That's untrue. That's just a thought and not a reality."*

"Thoughts lead to feelings; feelings lead to action. If you want to change how you feel, you have got to change how you think."

—DR. LAUREN

Everyone needs to have a daily routine and take care of themselves. Doing so allows us to radiate positive energy and beauty to the world.

MY PERSONAL TAKE

I was lucky that my life of constant movement forced me to both harness who I was and understand that we all have beauty in us. All we need to do is find it.

I am happy to say that although I have certain insecurities at times, I have found this beauty inside me through appreciating my *intangibles.*

I try to consciously practice *feeling* beautiful every day. When I say practice, I do mean practice because practice gets us closer to mastering a skill. Although this is not an exhaustive list, these are some of the things that are part of my inner beautifying daily routine.

No matter what happens throughout my week, or how crazy life gets I:

- Move my body four to five times a week
- Speak to my parents at least once a day
- Eat healthy and nutritious foods
- Put quality products on my skin (skin care and personal care is my "me" time)
- Surround myself with people who bring out the best in me
- Spend time with people I love
- Meet new people
- Learn new things

- Put myself out of my comfort zone at least once a day
- Do things that I enjoy
- Work on my passion projects
- Actively practice gratitude
- Actively practice positivity
- Sleep at least seven hours every night (some people need eight hours)

I am grateful that I can say I *feel* beautiful inside—well, most of the time. Doing all these things have really helped me be more mindful about my inner and outer beauty. As such, I encourage you to try out some that sound fitting for you. Unless you have already found a routine that works for you!

If you practice self-love, acceptance, confidence, and cultivation of inner beauty actively every day, you will become a true Master of it. People will be asking you left and right what you do to radiate such energy, and then you will be able to share the secret!

Having a routine—which could very well look completely different than mine—can help you be more self-aware, so you can distinguish between negative thoughts and facts. That little voice inside your head that often tries to trick you into going down the rabbit hole will become more distant and less present in your mind. When you realize you are having negative thoughts, you will be able to better push those thoughts away.

Such routines can help us protect ourselves from all the social and technological advancements in society that stimulate us on a daily basis. They can allow us to clear our mind and use these developments for good, rather than getting trapped in an online forum or odious thoughts about ourselves.

CHAPTER 8

POWER OF UNIQUE BEAUTY

———

"It's so important for you to find your power and beauty, that confidence within yourself. How do you find that confidence? By telling yourself that your flaws are what make you, you."

—PRIYANKA CHOPRA[237]

I would even say that what you may consider a flaw may be the most charming or endearing aspect of you to others.

———

237 Priyanka Chopra Jonas is an Indian actress, model, singer, and film producer who began her fame when she won the Miss World 2000 pageant.

Susana Martinez Vidal[238] agrees with this and says, "There is a huge error in overestimating perfection. Unique beauty makes you stand out from the crowd. That's why defects can be the most beautiful thing about you."

Yolanda Sacristán[239] adds to this idea and says:

> I feel very identified with the idea that imperfection makes you perfect. It is important to promote self-esteem and beauty instead of the traditional concepts of beauty homogenization that we have seen previously. Fortunately, today, beauty is understood from the idea of personality and diversity. We are beginning to verbally encourage the promotion of being unique. It invites us to embrace new forms of beauty.

We are bombarded by unattainable standards of beauty and what we are "supposed" to look like, maintaining a falsehood

---

238 Susana Martinez Vidal is a journalist and author, founder of *Ragazza* magazine, which catapulted her to becoming the youngest director of any edition of *Elle* in the world. After seeing the first exhibit of Frida Kahlo's clothing at the Casa Azul in 2012, she was inspired to write her first book, *Frida Kahlo: Fashion as the Art of Being*, recommended by *The New York Times* and *Vanity Fair* UK—most important magazines in more than twenty countries.

239 Yolanda Sactristán is the General Director of TheBeautyNewsroom. com and the former Editor-in-Chief of renowned publications: *Vogue* (2001-2017) and *Harper's Bazaar* (2017-2019). Yolanda is a skilled journalist with a passion for fashion, beauty, and luxury. She is always determined to produce compelling stories.

of perfection 24/7. This really means little to nothing because I can guarantee you that what is "perfect" for me is different than "perfect" for you.

Don't live through other people's validation. You should strive for your own acceptance.

JUST BE YOURSELF

"Beauty begins when you decide to be yourself."

—COCO CHANEL[240]

Frida Kahlo,[241] whose image is a true symbol of beauty still today, was never conventionally beautiful compared to the standards of her time, as Susana mentions. The commercialization of her image became one of the most renowned female symbols of natural and identity-based beauty, even though in many ways it was at odds with what she was trying to do with her art, which includes a profound reflection on suffering and trauma.

---

240 "A Quote by Coco Chanel." 2019. Goodreads.Com. Accessed October 6 2019. https://www.goodreads.com/quotes/7121021-beauty-begins-the-moment-you-decide-to-be-yourself.

241 Frida Kahlo (1907-1954) was a Mexican artist, activist and a deep political thinker, that was later through her art regarded as an icon for Chicanos, the feminist movement and the LGBT movement. Frida was known for her many portraits, self-portraits, and works inspired by nature and artifacts of Mexico.

Susana, the Kahlo connoisseur, stresses the importance of having a unique beauty like the one Frida expressed. "Frida was able to turn around her 'defects,' thick unibrow and mustache, and incorporate them into her own 'look' and her brand. They made her identity. "Frida Kahlo made her natural features into the essence of beauty itself, giving her name Frida Kahlo an aura of perpetual confidence that still resonates today," Susana elloquently notes.

Beauty goes far deeper than your image. It's the way you carry yourself, your identity, and your personality. Beauty is intangible.

Believe in yourself and be proud of who you are inside and out.

"Life is too short to suffer. Pain is inevitable, but suffering is optional. Don't take yourself too seriously. Love your uniqueness and your authentic quirks. Learn to dance with life a little."

—SUSANA MARTINEZ VIDAL

In *Ageless Beauty the French Way*, Clémence von Mueffling[242] quotes, "What is not perfect can sometimes be charming,

---

242 Clémence von Mueffling is the Founder and Editor of Beauty and Well-Being (BWB), which brings a fresh aesthetic to the beauty and well-being media. She is also the author of *Ageless Beauty the French Way*, a luxurious, entertaining, unparalleled guide to every French beauty secret for all women.

and what is already perfect does not need to be overdone."[243] Clémence continues by saying, "Going to any extreme in a vain search for 'perfection' will never leave anyone satisfied."[244] We should really tattoo that onto our hands and look at it every day.

We respect these ideas in theory but don't practice them quite enough. I'm sure it is not the first time you have heard this. However, it is key to repeat it to yourself often because we live in a society that is obsessed with perfection.

Thinking like this happens to the best of us, Klara Chrzuszcz[245] says.

> A phrase I often hear from my patients is "I want perfect skin." Since everyone has a different perception of perfection, I try to dive a little deeper to really understand what their ultimate goals are. From there we work together to get as close as we can to their goal. As we all know, there is no such thing as perfect

---

243 Mueffling, C. (n.d.). *Ageless Beauty the French Way*. 1st ed. New York City: St. Martin's Press, 2018. p.14.

244 Ibid.

245 Klara Chrzuszcz is a Medical Skin care Aesthetician, Clinical Skin care Expert, and the owner of Klara Beauty Lab. Klara is an educator in Europe for neurotoxin application as well as dermal fillers for the face and body, and she travels to teach on a yearly basis. Her approach involves delving into clients' lifestyles, diets, stress levels, etc. which, allows her to create a one-of-a-kind experience.

and I do believe the word is used more loosely than meaningfully. I think a better statement to say would be "I want the best skin I could possibly have," which is much more attainable and feasible. We can all be the best version of ourselves. And it is my job to help my patients get there.

OWN IT

Chinwe Esimai[246] moved from Nigeria to the US at the age of seventeen. You have read a part of her story in the previous chapter, and here is another anecdote that further accentuates the importance of owning your culture, your identity, and your uniqueness.

She recounts:

> When I moved to the US from Nigeria, there were moments when I questioned: *Am I good enough?* People would tell me I had a very "striking look" or that my cheekbones were so defined. These made me wonder:
>
> *Is it a bad thing to be that different? Is it a good thing?*

---

246 Chinwe Esimai is the Managing Director and Chief Anti-Bribery Officer at Citigroup, Inc. She is also an award-winning lawyer, author, and speaker who is passionate about inspiring generations of immigrant women leaders.

Do I even want to stand out this much?

Embracing my physical beauty has come with embracing my whole self. Over time, I've developed confidence with my work, confidence with my own experiences, and a deep understanding that embracing who I am and the uniqueness I bring—physically and otherwise—is really the best gift I can give to myself and to the world.

Now raising an eleven-year-old daughter, it is important for me to emphasize to her that beauty is more than what you see on the surface and we need to embrace what is unique and different in others.

We must view culture and identity not as something that separates us from society but as something positive that can bring, as Chinwe says, "magic to the conversation." It brings a different perspective and a new outlook to people.

EXPRESS YOURSELF, USE THAT INNER CREATIVITY

Expressing oneself is one of an individual's most natural instincts, whether it be through fashion, art, music, dance, writing, speaking, etc. Beauty is the incredible outcome of this expression. Sometimes it takes time to find what you're most comfortable with, but experiment until you find what makes you feel at ease and natural.

The importance of your personal quest is underrated especially when you come from two distinct backgrounds or more. As someone who grew up as a citizen of the world, I don't know if I would have had such a strong sense of identity if it weren't for ballet. This was my form of expression. No matter what country or city I lived in, ballet has allowed me to *feel* beautiful inside and out. Currently, I still hold on tightly to that form of beauty in my day-to-day and embody much of what I learned from my formative years dancing and my experiences on stage. I am forever thankful to the arts for making this quest attainable for me at such a young age.

Jordana Shiau,[247] a Chinese American woman who grew up in Los Angeles, expressed an interesting account of her experience with her own quest for beauty with two prominent and distinct cultures in her life.

> I think I have an interesting perspective because I feel like Western and Eastern standards of beauty are quite different. I grew up with conflicting ideals of

---

247 Jordana Shiau is a Manager of Social and Digital Strategy at Laura Mercier. She has been in the corporate side of the beauty industry for the last five years working from startups to the largest beauty brands in the world.

what was supposed to be beautiful, especially living in LA and having Asian parents. I loved being in the sun, tanning, going to the beach, and getting highlights in my hair. This was very different from the ideal of Eastern beauty, which I was exposed to at home.

My parents are from Taiwan, and ancestrally from China. They moved to the US in the '70s. As a result, I grew up with confined Asian beauty standards in my household. This was composed of having fair skin, almond shaped eyes, a thin nose, a nice pointy chin, and shiny black hair. I remember growing up, my mom would tell me, "Oh, your skin is so fair. It's so beautiful." (She's tanner than I am, and she always wished her skin was fairer.) She was always telling me to keep my skin fair and to stay away from the sun. I know my mother always meant well but it was a constant struggle for me because I had two very different standards of beauty between the one I saw with my friends and the one in my household.

As I grew up, I had to go on a quest to find my own perception of beauty, which interestingly aligns with neither of these two.

As I've gotten older, I've stopped trying to adhere to a certain standard of beauty. I have become more appreciative of what I have naturally. I can express myself in order to *feel* like myself.

I think moving away from LA, now living in New York, starting a career, and having my own separate life has made it a lot easier for me to define my own sense of beauty and what I *feel* comfortable in.

Experimenting with coloring my hair was something I love, so I do that now. My mom, surprisingly, is okay with it—I literally have bright orange hair—and so is my dad actually. There are still some limits, however. I can never get tattoos and I can never get piercings. The reason I can't get these is not because I don't want to but because a certain level of guilt comes with being a child of immigrant parents and knowing how much they sacrificed to get you where you are. I try not to be disrespectful to them. For them, tattoos and piercings are not a form of expression but more of a sign of disrespect. They perceive it as tarnishing your body.

I am an expressive person, but there are certain things I would not do because I have respect for my elders, which from my Asian background. It makes me *feel* beautiful to express myself enough, yet still respect my parents.

Respecting one's culture is also a form of beauty, not only for ourselves but for others. There is a unique beauty in people who abide by certain values brought by their culture.

HAVE FUN WITH IT

Mi Anne Chan,[248] who also comes from an Asian background, has found her quest of expression through colorful makeup, building a large following on YouTube and Instagram by sharing her unique beauty with others.

> I wear makeup almost every day. I came to a point years ago where I decided that if I was going to wear makeup, I was going to have fun with it, regardless of what people say. That's when I started experimenting with colors, textures, and finishes. Then I realized that a lot of women and men love talking about and engaging with makeup. It was a conversation starter, and it allowed me to connect with my audience, readers, and friends more intimately. I started putting it on Instagram to create a community. I absolutely love devouring makeup content on Instagram, so I thought I might as well give it a try

---

248 Mi Anne Chan is an Associate Producer and Staff Writer at Refinery29, a video director at Condé Nast entertainment, and a beauty influencer/ vlogger. She has been writing, editing, filming, and making tutorials on all things beauty related since the start of her career.

too. I love videos of makeup tutorials and very close macro-shots of pigments being applied to fresh skin.

Expressing yourself, like Mi Anne with makeup, can completely change the way you feel and even allow you to have some fun! Because why not revive the little kid inside us.

I don't wear much makeup in my everyday routine, but I still have an incredible relationship with makeup as a form of expression. The spectacular feeling of being on stage dancing, my solo in *Swan Lake* with my full face of stage makeup on is an unimaginable feeling. I can perfectly picture my swan costume, the lights shooting directly on my face, and all the sea of little heads staring at me from a distance in the crowd. This is how I best expressed myself for years. This specific moment was probably one of the times I felt most beautiful.

CAN YOU MAINTAIN YOUR UNIQUE BEAUTY WITH COSMETIC TREATMENTS OR PROCEDURES?

Short answer. Yes.

Actually, most of the best of plastic surgeons and leading dermatologists in the world, including the ones I spoke to, refuse to do work on patients who request to look anything other than an enhanced version of themselves. Procedures and treatments can be tremendously helpful in making insecurities or abnormalities fade away. It is incredible to know procedures out there can positively affect someone's life dramatically, making them more confident in every part of their life. Confidence can open literal doors.

Dr. Sami Helou[249] said:

> We are finding ourselves not with a very similar standard of beauty. When an actress, model, or someone of influence launches a new look, everyone wants to imitate it. For example, all over the world there is a lot of excess on how people do lips because that is what people want now. There is a tendency to do more than needed. But this is not only on the patient and what the patient is asking for. If the patient wants an unnatural and exaggerated look, it's up to the doctor to guide them in the correct direction. It is almost more important for the doctor to have a pointed professional awareness in order to perform on their patients a proportional and elegant enhancement. They need to have an esthetic respect to the unique beauty of the person. In my opinion this is where the real problem lies. Many doctors don't have this and do their job with no professionalism, or just for the money so they do what the patient asks for.

249 Dr. Sami Helou is one of the most renowned specialized plastic surgeons in Beirut, Lebanon.

The role of the doctor is to guide the patient because they are the professionals and the ones who should know what aesthetically looks proper on a patient.

It's a privilege to have such an array of technologies, treatments, and cosmetic procedures that can make it more affordable and feasible to enhance features that might have a significant impact on the way one feels. For cosmetic adjustments, it is important to prioritize how you *feel* and not how you look. For this reason, it becomes imperative to have the best hands do your work, if you are looking to get "something done."

The best doctors will encourage you to do only what is needed and not more.

Don't try to fix what is not broken.

NO NEED FOR A MIRROR

Twenty years ago, if you wanted to see your own reflection you had to scout a glass window, step into a bathroom, or hope that one of your friends had a small makeup mirror in their purse. Now it's as easy as looking down at your phone. Mediums like Snapchat, Instagram, Facetime, Skype, etc... just add to it.

All of this exposure to our self-image makes us more critical than we would have ever been about every aspect of our faces.

As a consequence, our insecurities take deeper roots. No one likes to be constantly reminded of something they don't like, especially when it is about themselves; with the lives we live today we see reflections an unhealthy amount.

Face-tune, photoshop, filters, and similar apps that can "enhance" our appearance have unfortunately caused a heightened demand for procedures. Generation Zers and millennials who really manipulate these apps have a vision of what they would like to look like—out of mere practice. Lara Devgan, a board-certified plastic surgeon in New York City, spoke to *Allure* magazine and said, "Now, people want to look more like their own filtered photos or a Photoshop version of themselves. And recently, people are super into the tiny little micro-optimizations that make them feel a little bit more confident but are not completely obvious."[250]

For this reason, it is easier for them to want to look like that IRL and thus, some turn to plastic surgery, fillers, laser, and other treatments. It is not bad to turn to these if you have a healthy mindset about them. But unfortunately, lots of people who go this route want to fill a void that a cosmetic adjustment will never be able to remedy in the long run.

---

250 Nast, Condé. 2019. "The 7 Plastic Surgery Trends That Will Be Huge This Year." *Allure*. Accessed November 6 2019. https://www.allure.com/story/plastic-surgery-procedure-trends-2019.

If someone can *feel* more beautiful by enhancing their own unique beauty, this is always a plus. Before, women more often came in with photographs of models or actresses that looked nothing like them, wanting to have surgery to get a closer appearance to whomever it was. The line is excessively thin between wanting a "tweakment" and going into a spiral of feeling like every one of your quirks is a defect while each one can be your most charming features. [251]

On the other hand, as Dr. Sami Helou says:

> The dysmorphophobia pathology, characterized by obsession with an imaginary defect, whose perception of the person is completely disproportionate, is found everywhere now. I see women all the time who have magnificent lips but want to get them done. They get them enhanced but they don't think they are done enough and then they end up looking like a caricature.

Dr. Helou is talking about an excess that makes you lose your unique beauty. "To be focused on your external appearance so much so that you allow what you look like to dictate your self-worth will only go so far before you realize that physical alterations are not the answer," Sami Helou says.

---

251 Nast, Condé. 2019. "The 7 Plastic Surgery Trends That Will Be Huge This Year." *Allure.* Accessed November 6 2019. https://www.allure.com/story/plastic-surgery-procedure-trends-2019.

When one undergoes an excessive change to their face, they end up looking like nothing at all. This is when all uniqueness disappears.

MORE ACCESSIBLE THAN EVER

Innovation in formulations and cutting-edge technology have allowed cosmetic enhancements to be more inclusive, more available, and accessible to everyone. As *Allure* mentions, "Injectables, like Botox and fillers, have become so mainstream that, according to the American Academy of Facial Plastic and Reconstructive Surgery (AAFPRS)'s annual survey, four-fifths of all treatments performed by facial plastic surgeons in 2018 were cosmetic, non-surgical procedures, thanks to the subtle but noticeable results and relatively reasonable cost."[252]

Many noninvasive options such as injectables, lasers, and treatments take very little time to get done and have very quick recovery rates. People can now go in and out with barely any downsides. These are a lot more affordable too, which is making it more attainable for people from all socio-economic classes. According to the American Society of Plastic Surgeons, minimally invasive cosmetic procedures

252 Nast, Condé. 2019. "The 7 Plastic Surgery Trends That Will Be Huge This Year." *Allure*. Accessed October 3 2019. https://www.allure.com/story/plastic-surgery-procedure-trends-2019.

have grown nearly 200 percent since 2000, and they don't look to be slowing down anytime soon.[253]

When speaking about this with Klara Chrzuszcz,[254] she told me, "More women are having what I call the 'Fifth Avenue Syndrome,' the explosion of plastic surgery and fillers amongst affluent women in NYC; so many don't look natural anymore. When there is an addiction to surgery, it is the doctor's job to guide or stop them to help them. It is their job to care for the patient and not just perform surgeries and treatments for the profit."

We want to avoid this at all costs. First, focus on finding your beauty from within. Then, let your urge to get something "done" sit in your brain for a while. And then, if you would like to go with an enhancement a year or two years later, go for it. Make sure you have deeply researched the doctor, the procedures and all the options out there before letting anyone touch your face. Using this method of first inner, then outer can save you from cosmetic disasters that are simply unnecessary.

Dr. Devgan, a board-certified plastic surgeon in New York City supports this, telling *Allure* magazine, "It's really the

---

253 Ibid.

254 Klara Chrzuszcz is a Medical Skin care Aesthetician, Clinical Skin care Expert, and the owner of Klara Beauty Lab. Klara is an educator in Europe for neurotoxin application as well as dermal fillers for the face and body, and she travels to teach on a yearly basis. Her approach involves delving into clients' lifestyles, diets, stress levels, etc. which, allows her to create a one-of-a-kind experience.

era of minimally invasive medical aesthetic procedures."[255] I think that is not only because of low downtime, lower cost, and lower invasiveness, but also because there's lower stigma and lower barrier to entry."

According to Dr. Devgan, "micro-optimizations," as she categorizes them, "include the unorthodox use of filler in locations other than the traditional cheekbone, like the earlobe to tighten a stretched piercing from heavy earrings, or the bridge of the nose during a noninvasive rhinoplasty."[256]

Cosmetic noninvasive enhancements are more inclusive to all skin tones and genders as well. Dr. Julian Few[257] mentions on *The Beauty Closet* by Goop podcast, that innovation in fillers and treatments along with the possibility of stacking these treatments[258] better enhances your face without surgery.[259] Cosmetic surgery in the past had been a subject of worry for people of color due to scaring, as each skin type

255 Nast, Condé. 2018. "Everything You've Ever Wanted To Know About Fillers." *Allure*. Accessed October 3 2019. https://www.allure.com/story/facial-fillers-information-guide.

256 Ibid.

257 Dr. Julian Few is the Founder, The Few Institute for Aesthetic Plastic Surgery.

258 Stacking treatments refers to doing many noninvasive treatments at once to amplify the result.

259 "Dr. Few: A Plastic Surgeon On Going Little (Not Big) | Goop." 2019. *Goop*. Accessed November 6 2019. https://goop.com/beauty-closet-podcast/dr-few-a-plastic-surgeon-on-going-little-not-big/.

scars differently. Stacking these treatments is something Dr. Few loves to do for results that seem to look as effective as surgery but are less expensive and more accessible for all of us diverse busy bees.

In terms of gender, Dr. Lara Devgan says that about fifteen percent of her patients are male, and that number has been increasing dramatically. She constitutes this rise of male patients to a demand for more classically masculine features, and the looser taboo on getting cosmetic procedures.[260] Dr. Devgan explains, "A lot of the procedures that I'm doing enhance features to look more masculine. Men have historically been interested in the lower third of the face, meaning the chin, neck, and jawline," and now they are easily achievable.[261]

What Top Things Do People Want to get Done in General?

I asked Dr. John Martin[262] this question and he answered with a few things that are now very *à la mode*:

260 Nast, Condé. 2019. "The 7 Plastic Surgery Trends That Will Be Huge This Year." *Allure*. Accessed October 3 2019. https://www.allure.com/story/plastic-surgery-procedure-trends-2019.

261 Ibid.

262 Dr. John Martin is a Harvard-educated Medical Doctor who specializes in Facial Cosmetic Surgery as well as other non-surgical treatment for vascular and pigment problems as well as skinrejuvenation. Dr. Martin has been featured in *The Doctors, The Dr. Oz Show, Dr. Phil,* and *Anderson Cooper 360°*.

- **Neurotoxins:** Botox, Disport etc. These are the most common things people want even at a young age. They are a great way to decrease lines around the eyes and forehead with no downtime.

- **Fillers:** Non-surgical way to improve appearance—adding volume to plump up areas that have lost volume as we age.

- **Energy devices:** Laser, radiofrequency, ultrasound. Non-surgical way to tighten skin and improve skin texture, often without much downtime.

THREE MAIN CONSUMERS

Many trends are developing in today's world of fast communication. There are also three general consumer types: The "Extreme Makeover," the "All Natural," and the "Make Me Look Natural" individuals. All of these tend to gravitate more toward some trends than others. These *three consumer types* are very prominent, and almost everyone falls under one or another.

Which one do you fall under?

None of these categories are anything to be proud or ashamed of, and each has its own powerful way of making us *feel* beautiful.

**The following are three generalizations I have picked up on during my research.

The "Extreme Makeover" Individual

This individual leans toward more aggressive and repetitive cosmetic procedures. They are mostly centered on the medical aspect of beauty and want to see big results and fast. Many of these individuals usually remain unsatisfied with their physical appearance and reach for more in order to compensate. Some, not all, of the people who fall under this category are obsessed with their outward appearance and typically start to resemble each other.

The All-Natural Individual

This individual is likely to never dip their toes into the cosmetic procedures pool but will use some natural and clean beauty products to make sure they stay as naturally beautiful as they can. The "no-makeup look" has been very much adopted by many individuals of this group as this presents a better version of their real selves. This trend has brought individuals to accept their beauty as it is—authentic and unique, without camouflage.[263]

---

263 "Why More Women Are Happily Going Without Makeup." 2019. *Psychology Today.* Accessed October 3 2019. https://www.psychologytoday.com/ca/blog/the-clarity/201707/why-more-women-are-happily-going-without-makeup.

The "Make Me Look Natural" Individual

This individual tends to fall somewhere in the middle of the former two as they are willing to go through some cosmetic procedures and treatments to enhance their features but always while remaining true to their unique beauty. The people who fall in this broad middle spectrum are harder to specify, but they are more willing to conform to some trends because they are more moldable on one side or the other. They would be willing to experiment with products from the medical and potent side and ones on the more natural side as well. These middle individuals can also decide to go to either extreme sides.

"Doctor, Make It look Natural Please"

Many more people are requesting minimally invasive procedures for a more "natural look." This is the trending look at the moment, according to Dr. Helou. Just like the "no-makeup makeup look." Dr. Helou says, "I have started seeing more of a 'natural look' trend coming back after years of so much exaggeration."

He thinks people from all races and backgrounds around the world are doing the same procedures, which is making them begin to resemble each other. "It is maybe not a conscious effort to look all the same, but more like the consequence of what they do that makes them look all the same," says Dr.

Helou. For this reason, he believes the perception of beauty is becoming more reasonable and more representative of what people look like all over the world and therefore leaning toward a more "natural look" approach, to avoid everyone looking the same.

THE SHIFT FROM REPARATIVE TO PREVENTATIVE

Now, a much younger demographic is starting to indulge in cosmetics. A desire of always needing to look "perfect" because of social media has caused younger generations to make appointments with surgeons and clinical dermatologists to "fix" the way they look. They frequently make their appointments themselves, with the consent of their parents, as Klara noted.

Preventative cosmetic treatments are booming. The demographic is not only older individuals who want to enhance their features to correct some of the effects of age anymore. We have now a whole other group of consumers who want to get enhancements to get a certain "look." This is very controversial in the cosmetic world because some doctors approve preventative measures, and others like some I have interviewed believe it is not necessary to act on "flaws" that do not exist. According to a professional in the medical aesthetic industry,[264] the earlier young adults begin participating in preventative measures, the more hooked they will get to the quick fix approach as they grow older.

The medical aesthetic industry professional pointed out something very interesting: a new marketing strategy going on in doctor offices and dermatology consultations. There have recently been more and more advertisements for preventative measures for young patients in the waiting rooms of clinical treatment centers. This marketing strategy is directed at parents, but generally mothers who are getting treatments themselves, so they are inclined to bring their teenagers or twenty-year-olds to the office. These sons and daughters of patients who come in, most likely millennials or Generation Zers, are called, "Industry Darlings," which means they begin young in the cosmetic enhancement world and stay in it forever. It becomes normal for them to continue getting enhancements done since they were exposed to the industry at such a young age.

This professional believes it is completely unnecessary to get Botox before you need it. Young women, however, are starting to believe they should be getting Botox to prevent fine lines and wrinkles when is no need. This professional pointed out

---

264 This industry professional wishes to keep personal and company information anonymous.

how people are now losing the beauty of human expression because of the overuse of these kinds of injectables.

Dr. Sami Helou says, "I think Botox for prevention without having any wrinkles is like taking antibiotics before you are sick, which I find incorrect."

"You can give maintenance and prevention to your skin through beauty rituals. Make them part of your life, of your daily routine and this will show results and help you feel more self-confident. If you feel like you feel good, you will be looking good and turning that into self-confidence."

—A PROFESSIONAL IN THE MEDICAL
AESTHETIC INDUSTRY[265]

Nayera Senane,[266] who specializes in everything that has to do with lips, says, "Five years ago I had predominantly older female patients, but now, I have a lot of younger patients who want to look like someone else. I get a lot less corrective work and more preventative or enhancement work." Of course, corrective cosmetics will always be an enormous part of the market,

---

265 This industry professional wishes to keep personal and company information anonymous.

266 Nayera Senane is a Diamond Allergan Injector, Botox and dermal filler expert. She currently holds a wide client base including celebrities and models. Although based in Los Angeles, she travels regularly to the East Coast to see clients.

especially now that we are living so much longer. But the market of preventative cosmetics is emerging at an incredibly fast pace.

Most doctors and clinical dermatologists I have spoken to agree that the best way to approach preventative measures are by taking care of your skin and approaching it with a more holistic approach to beauty.

HOOKED ON "THE LOOK"

A movement has begun with our society's perception of what is beautiful, but there is still a long way to go. Places like South Korea seem to be going in the opposite direction of natural. Their beauty icons are almost all the ones who have been surgically reconstructed. They have double eyelids,[267] thinned noses, pointier chins, higher cheekbones, and more, affirmed a Generation Z beauty connoisseur and university student and influencer from Hong Kong.[268]

In South Korea and some parts of China, there is a sense of maturity in getting a facial reconstruction or at least the double-eyelid surgery. Somewhere between the eighteenth and twenty-ninth birthday, women tend to get a facial enhancement to look like

---

267 A double eyelid is a crease of the skin over the eyes. People in Asia frequently get surgery to get this crease.
268 This industry professional wishes to keep personal and company information anonymous.

a lot of KOLs they follow, as the HK influencer explained. For many young girls, this is a step closer toward reaching beauty.

"We are a collective society, so the more people begin to invest in a product or treatment, the more everyone else will want to as well," says the beauty connoisseur and influencer from HK.[269] Contrary to popular belief, Asians are not getting cosmetic surgery to look more "Westernized." They get these surgeries to look like "more beautiful Asians," which is different, Li Binbin, a Beijing-based plastic surgeon, explained to the *South China Morning Post*.[270] "In the East, we have our own beauty standards," Binbin says.[271]

Beauty in the region is very heavily influenced by Korean Pop, or K-pop, as many entertainers within the industry have all gone through facial reconstructions themselves. Hence, it is hard for the standard of beauty that is influenced in China or on girls in South Korea to ever be met unless they go through a facial enhancement themselves. The South Korean beauty standard is specifically strict and not only does it set the tone for beauty in South Korea, but it also has an enormous

---

269 Person has requested not to disclose their name for personal reasons.

270 "The Angelababy Effect: More Women Want Double Eyelid Like Actress." 2017. *South China Morning Post*. Accessed October 3 2019. https://www.scmp.com/lifestyle/health-beauty/article/2093921/why-double-eyelid-surgery-rise-asia-rising-incomes-and.

271 Ibid.

influence on the Chinese public and on Asia's beauty market as a whole, making *feeling* beautiful quite a hard task.

SIGNATURE FEATURE

Let's talk about Dr. Shamban's Signature Feature concept from chapter 1 of this book.

First, Dr. Shamban says it is incredible how many people are unclear of what their Signature Feature is. By the way, I was one of those.

Dr. Shamban says:

> When I give a talk about Signature Feature at conventions or conferences, which I have given at least ten in different countries around the world, I always stop when describing what Signature Feature[272] and I make everyone turn to the person next to them and tell them what their Signature Feature is. It should be done in a blink. It's a subcortical kind of thing that you find subconsciously at first glance.

When she told me this, of course, I had to ask Dr. Shamban what mine was! She suggested they were my eyes, which was

---

272 Signature Feature means something about your face that is very compelling and memorable.

crazy to hear given I had never thought anything special of my eyes before. This proved to me that I don't see myself the same way as others see me. It is shocking how unaware we can be of how other people perceive us.

In general, it is good to know what your Signature Feature is, so you can be aware of your uniqueness and cherish it.

Do it yourself! Ask anyone around you, even a stranger, what the most memorable feature of your face is, and you will be surprised. Then make sure you are aware of it, so you can use it to your advantage.

For example, since now I know for me it's my eyes, I pay more attention to them. I am more aware of my eyes when speaking to people. Once you know about your Signature Feature, it becomes something you can hold on to and something that is key to your identity.

"No matter what happens, if you're thin, if you're overweight, if you're young, if you're old, if you're rich, if you're poor, if you are challenged in any way, you still have your Signature Feature," said Dr. Shamban.

Dr. Shamban further elaborates:

It's usually eyes or mouth because those are the central features of your face, but in some cases, it can be someone's hair, or it could be off the face such as waist, bottom or breast.

My patients just want to look their best. When they come to me, they know my reputation and they know I will not do anything on them that wouldn't look good on them, even if they asked me to. But they don't usually ask me to do something I would not approve of anyways because they know my philosophy. I only clear the canvas, or what I call "background noise." It's not about changing any features. It's about allowing the eye to see the important ones. I'll just tell them what I'm going to do to them, and my clients trust me. But if they did ask me for anything that I think would not enhance their authentic beauty, I would say, "Sorry, I am not the right doctor for you."

Dr. Alouie also[273] relates her success to make her patients feel beautiful through pointing out their unique features. This allows her patients to feel better and really transmit their inner beauty.

---

273 Dr. Jouhayna Alouie is a well-known esthetician in Beirut, Paris, and Riyadh, who has been working in the field since the mid-seventies. She specializes in corrective work, permanent makeup, and enhancement facial treatments. In the past, she has worked closely with Miss France and many Arab celebrities.

Dr. Alouie says:

> I start by focusing on the patient's beauty assets and then I address what can be done to enhance or highlight those assets. By using this approach, the patient feels more beautiful without losing her unique personality. I help her develop her own unique beauty style. In a way, I help her develop to her own beauty potential. From my experience, my patients feel beautiful when they feel confident and satisfied with the results. This requires carefully listening to my patients, appreciating their sensitivities so I can develop an appropriate assessment, communicating clearly my plan with my patient, and executing the plan with the highest level of skills.

There's only one of you. There's never ever going to be another person like you. So that is the power of unique beauty in and of itself. Make decisions that make sense for your beauty. You need to know yourself and cultivate that beauty from within first.

CHAPTER 9

THREE BEAUTIES MAKING A DIFFERENCE IN A SECTOR THEY DIDN'T EXPECT

———

Three women I had the honor to spend time with during my research for this book have forever made an imprint on my life. Beyond just me, these three women have impacted countless individuals around the globe with their drive, passion, tenacity, and continued hard work. The beauty industry is forever marked by Jeanette Sarkisian Wagner,[274] Anastasia Soare,[275] Dr. Barbara Sturm.[276]

These radiant, humble, confident, and authentic women have fully conquered their beauty from within. I am enlightened by them and I hope you will be too.

JEANETTE WAGNER

"I do not want us to be the biggest. I want us to be the best. *Nulli Secundus*: Second to None."

—JEANETTE WAGNER

274 Jeanette Wagner is the Vice Chairman Emerita of The Estée Lauder Companies Inc. Mrs. Wagner joined the Estée Lauder Companies as the Vice President, Director of Marketing of the Estée Lauder brand in the International Division. In that role, she revolutionized the process of bringing products to market and exploded the growth of the Lauder brand internationally. She is also Chairman CEO of Nulli Secundus Associates, a pro bono consulting company.

275 Anastasia Soare is the founder, CEO, and driving force behind Anastasia Beverly Hills—one of the fastest-growing brands in the beauty industry. In 1990, she introduced a new brow shaping technique to clients—later patented as the Golden Ratio Eyebrow Shaping Method—that has gone on to become a modern beauty essential. Anastasia is a beauty pioneer and powerhouse.

276 Dr. Barbara Sturm is the founder and CEO of Dr. Barbara Sturm Molecular Cosmetics. She is a German aesthetics doctor, widely renowned for her anti-inflammatory philosophy and her non-surgical anti-aging skin treatments. Dr. Sturm translated science from her clinical research and orthopedic practice into the field of aesthetics and has been a success ever since.

Jeanette Wagner has been named one of the most inspirational women not only in the United States but all over the world. She has spent her life doing what she does best, taking an idea or story with a strong identity and adapting it to other cultures, countries, and regions of the world.

Who is the Smartest Person You Know?

Jeanette grew up in an Armenian family of immigrants to the US after the genocide. She grew up during The Great Depression with no recollection of ever seeing any cosmetics in the house. In high school, her idea of a full face of makeup was walking out of the house with lipstick on.

All her life, Jeanette loved writing and wanted to become a journalist. She worked for the Walgreen Company as an editor and went on to become an editor for the *Chicago Daily News* weekly magazine, leading her to be the first female editor of the *Saturday Evening Post*. Years later, Jeanette was lured to *Cosmopolitan Magazine* to be their articles editor.

An interesting opportunity came along for Jeanette because Hearst Corporation wanted to invest in an international division, creating *Cosmopolitan* in each language in over a dozen countries in Europe, Asia, and Africa. They asked Jeanette to be the Editorial Director of the International Division. So solid was the foundation set forth by Jeanette that the division remains the corporation's most profitable arm. This global experience eventually led to her success at Estée Lauder, allowing her to make her mark on the beauty industry.

Jeanette explains:

> The trick was how do you keep the DNA of a magazine that is uniquely American and at the same launch it in Africa, England, Spain, France, and over a dozen countries to meet the wants/needs of the local readers. I had a global view of the world, so I knew how to take the DNA and adapt it so it could resonate with the "Cosmo Girl" in Spain, in England, etc... without turning into something quite different.
>
> At the same time Leonard Lauder had a small international business he wanted to grow. He felt no one in his company could execute the assignment correctly to ship their US products overseas.

Leonard Lauder separately asked the two smartest women in his company who they considered to be the smartest person they knew, and they both gave him Jeanette's name. These two women were not special friends, yet both picked Wagner. Very intrigued, Mr. Lauder, asked Jeanette Wagner to lunch.

Jeanette at the time had been working for *Cosmo*. "I knew nothing about beauty, nor anything about the international business of beauty." I would disagree as Jeanette Wagner radiated beauty and excellence, the sort of charisma you look for in every leader when charting into unknown territories.

After a long lunch of questions about her life in journalism, Mr. Lauder proceeded to the most important part. "Before I met you I had a job in mind for you, but now that we've met, I see it's not a big enough position for you."

Jeanette Wagner: *"I thought, well isn't he gallant. He never wants to see me again, but he's paying me a compliment."*

Then Leonard Lauder said, "I need to organize my international division at Estée Lauder and when I do that, I will call you." I thought, *"I never expected to hear from him again. I was wrong!"*

Mr. Lauder did exactly that. The next day he offered her a job and she began her career at one of the most influential beauty houses in the world, turning their international division from the smallest and least profitable division to the largest and most profitable.

How did she do this? Jeanette was way ahead of her time.

Before globalization became the norm for big corporations, Jeanette was already brainstorming innovative strategies to bring actionable ideas to different regions of the world. Jeanette did her homework; she carefully went through every article that was published in international *Cosmo Magazines*, and she visited every country to meet and coach staff on *Cosmo's* DNA. She was very hands on.

"I didn't know anything about the international business of beauty. But, that's how I got into the business."

—JEANETTE WAGNER

Playing the Game by Her Rules

I want you to read it from her own words:

> I've given speeches about how a girl who knew nothing about cosmetics got hired by a major cosmetic company to build their international division and turned it from a small and least profitable division into the biggest and most profitable.
>
> Estée Lauder was an American company and privately held. Their idea was "We make it, you ship it" to the international division. They really had a mentality of "just sell what we make." Whereas,

my attitude was: think globally, and act locally in each country.

All the magazines we had inaugurated were made very successful because I had a sense of how to take something and keep its nature yet adapt it. You can do that if you understand globalization and cultural differences. Not only are the skin colors in these countries different but their mentalities are different. That understanding gave me the vision of how to take this company international. It meant changing a lot of rules and I got a lot of pushback.

On my very first day in the company, no one took me to lunch; I had no office. The man who was running Aramis International, a 6' 2" or more Englishman, came up to me on the first day and said: "I think it's ridiculous you're here. You should be home, having babies and taking care of your husband."

I started to laugh and in fact I could not stop laughing. A year later we were friends and he asked me to help him.

I got a lot of pushback from Domestic. They didn't want to do any of the things International was suggesting. They would not invite me to their meetings until one day Leonard Lauder went into one of the domestic meetings and looked around and didn't see me. He asked the head of the US Division, "Where is Jeanette?" and the answer was, "Oh, she was busy or something."

Then Leonard Lauder said, "Well, call her up and when she can come, I'll come back."

By doing that he definitely sent the message of "I'm paying attention to her and you better start paying attention to her too."

I looked at what they were doing in the few countries they were in, and whether Estée Lauder was meeting their corporate DNA as well as local needs. For example, in England, the best-selling lipsticks are pink shades, but in Germany the best-selling lipstick colors are in the orange shades. The company had a manufacturing standard minimum of 25,000 units to keep a color in the line. Since neither country was meeting its target quantities on some shades, many popular colors were cancelled.

We changed that. We analyzed every single country, and we looked at their needs, such as which color palettes worked best and what the right cream textures for their skin types were. We began to build and promote the brand with the kind of colors and the kind of skin care that suited those countries. Once we began including products in those countries that were designed with their consumer in mind, the brand gained international notoriety. This was the turning point where we saw sales go from small to huge increases. We opened Russia in 1989, China in 1992, and this put Estée Lauder ahead of the curve of any other major cosmetic company.

Do Your Homework

Jeanette continued:

This was happening because now we were doing our homework. We weren't just shipping any product made for the US.

That's my number one lesson. Do your homework.

You cannot do your homework sitting in the office in New York City. Visit every country before you ever think of launching a line. I learned this in the world of journalism.

What's the nature of their skin type?

What is the weather climate?

What are they selling?

What do they like?

Do they like fragrance?

Do they have fragrance?

In Japan, as you might know, you can't put fragrance in any skin care product. They really don't enjoy fragrance in their personal care products, and here we were sending products with fragrance in them. We had to start respecting that. So, Estée Lauder began manufacturing skin care products for Japan in special kettles in our Belgian plant where no products were manufactured. Again, business continued to grow.

Estée Lauder's motto was: "Every woman can be beautiful, and I will show you how." And that works in every country in the world. Our packaging was the same, our fashion was the same, but we changed how we looked at each country's consumer.

Changing the Perception of Beauty but Most Importantly of Life for a Society

Jeanette Wagner told a story that had me on my feet.

In the Soviet Union, which it was then, there were no perfumeries, per se. All real estate sites were controlled by the mayor of the city. We had a smart team at Estée Lauder that understood global negotiations and were experts on international business contracts. They scouted the first location for Estée Lauder in Moscow and thought they made a deal. The next thing we knew, one of our cosmetic competitors had stolen the space with some private contract. Three of us immediately flew to Moscow to see the competitor's location and though there were posters inside of their products, none of them were available to sell to customers. I found out all the products that were to have been sold in that store were going out the back door to all the wives of the heads of the Communist Party. I was happy the competitor had taken this location from us; it was a mediocre space and location. I learned several valuable lessons.

Stand by your values or don't do the deal.

I found the location I liked, right by the subway and right in the heart of Moscow. Now, I had to negotiate with the mayor. The mayor was happy to give me the location but wanted to sell Soviet Products in the mix as well. I said, "Excuse me, either I sell Estée Lauder products or no deal, and I really mean it." Millions of dollars were invested, but I was determined to walk away unless I got the deal that was right for Lauder. Rather than lose the whole contract, he said okay.

This was the time when the USSR was still having great shortages. People had to stand in seven-hour lines to buy primary food items like milk, bread, eggs, without knowing if there would be enough by the time they got to the front of the line. My vision was: In our stores we'll hand out a shopping list of products we have for sale inside to the customers standing in line, so they could check off what they wanted and hand it back to the sales staff once inside the store. This would ensure they got the products they wanted while reducing wait times. The sales-people would go up to the customer and say, "Yes, we have it! You will get what you have on your list! They were thrilled to know they'd receive the products they wanted. We also made our own shopping bags, all of which said Estée Lauder, which we gave away. It was nice advertising.

We exploded. We just exploded.

The mayor and I had a big disagreement about what percentage of Estée Lauder product we were going to have in the store. I wanted 100 percent and he wanted less than 50 percent. I said I wouldn't do it and I wouldn't sell at all if that was the case. I said if you're trying to prove things are getting better in the USSR, but only selling 50 percent or more of the products internationally, things aren't getting better. But, imagine what will happen if they get to the front of the line and they get the lipstick and they get the perfume they want. Now, things are getting better. This PR will be fantastic. So that's exactly what happened, and he agreed to keep it at 100 percent because it rebounded to his credit.

That's why you do your homework, you get deeply involved, you understand your consumers before you do anything, and you make sure that you're running a business that sticks to your DNA.

Jeanette is a genius with mission, vision, and drive. Although these stories are just a tiny highlight reel of what Jeanette did in her time in the beauty industry, I wanted to share with you the story of Estée Lauder entering the USSR because this was monumental. Upon hearing this story, I was on the brink of tears. I could not believe the talent of this woman, her ideas, and her capacity to understand other cultures without having lived in them. I spent six months in Russia and got to sense the feeling from people who lived through the time of shortages what they felt. I can only imagine what Estée Lauder abundance of beauty products could have done for women. In those hard times, beauty comes in as a "feel good" factor. A time to feel more beautiful when everything seems to be in disorder around you. Jeanette Wagner was able to make this happen for the women of Moscow.

Jeanette's legacy at Estée Lauder stretched beyond her own résumé. She made conscious decisions to uplift others. Jeanette said, "Aside from the few senior women (Estée Lauder and Evelyn Lauder,) a half dozen smart women were not being promoted to senior executive ranks." Jeanette focused on the importance of brains and abilities. During her time there, she was able to bring awareness and attention to overlooked talent within the company and develop the smartest people worldwide, both male and female.

"You were the toughest boss I ever had, the best boss I ever had. I never learned so much. And I never had a better time."
—PEOPLE WHO WORKED FOR JEANETTE WAGNER

ANASTASIA SOARE

Anastasia Soare is one of the most successful, self-made businesswomen in the world, with an eponymous beauty brand valued at an estimated $3 billion. A single mother and immigrant from Romania, Anastasia didn't even speak the language when she arrived in the United States in 1989. Three decades later, she's built an empire. Anastasia beat the odds and overcame all obstacles to get where she is today by putting eyebrows—the modern-day beauty essential—on the map.

It all began when Anastasia was working as an esthetician, a job she was able to acquire without being proficient in English. Responsible for facials and waxing, she noticed something peculiar.

> While working at the salon, I realized nobody really paid much attention to their eyebrows. Nobody shaped them, and they were a complete afterthought, if they were even considered at all. At some point, a lightbulb went off, and I remembered my art teacher instructing us that if you wanted to change the emotion of a portrait, all you had to change were the eyebrows. Around this time, I had started working with quite a few celebrity clients (Cindy Crawford, Oprah Winfrey, Naomi Campbell, Faye Dunaway, Jennifer

Lopez, among others), and they became the earliest adopters of my developing brow shaping technique.

By 1996, Anastasia found herself exclusively devoted to brows. While shaping the infinitely varied arches that walked through her door, she recognized another thing missing from the market—eyebrow products. With a little ingenuity, Anastasia would create her own mixture of eyeshadow, Vaseline, and Aloe Vera to create a pomade with which she would fill in the overall shape of clients' brows after waxing. Three weeks later, the clients would be back, saying how they loved their brows when immediately leaving the salon, but after washing their faces they could see the gaps created from over-tweezing. Anastasia knew she had to create something her clients could take with them and use at home. She knew it was time to start creating a product line exclusively for brows—the first of its kind.

I Got It from My Mother

Anastasia recounts:

My mother used to make clothes for women in Romania. Clients would come to the shop and peruse a thick catalogue, selecting their looks and a fabric before my mother would get to work creating it from scratch. Communism gripped the country, and during that time there was nothing you could go and simply buy from a department store. If you wanted something, it had to be made to order.

As I did my homework between the sewing machines, I learned to become my mother's eyes and began to sketch dresses for her clients. I watched as she took a client's measurements: the arms, hips, and the chest. She nipped, tucked, and adjusted, her eye intuitively fixated on the importance of balance and proportion. I remember her saying, "When you draw this dress, take care to balance her silhouette. Since her shoulders are small relative to her hips, add upper structure and shoulder pads to create the correct proportion."

My mother wasn't professionally trained, nor could she put a name to this principle of thirds she was upholding, but her eye instinctively sensed this need for balance and proportion when fitting clothing onto a wide variety of body types. At the same time in school, I was learning about the concept of the Golden Ratio. Also referred to as Divine Proportion, it was naturally occurring in nature, had influenced centuries of art and architecture, and had even been used by the likes of Leonardo da Vinci.

I didn't know it at the time, but this combined training would become invaluable when I turned my focus to the faces of clients years later. Suddenly, it all clicked. What I had learned in school, the way my mother had trained my eye on bodies—not only was it all connected, but also, I could continue the story with a revolutionary way of shaping brows.

My mother was beloved and in demand by so many. Growing up in her shop taught me one more invaluable lesson about being a business owner: always put the client first. Through the long hours, large orders, and sheer volume of people who would walk through the door, my mother made each feel like a friend. She was widely respected not only for her talent, but for how she treated people. I never forgot that, and because of her, fostering relationships has always been a top priority in my career. I have had clients for thirty years who still come back.

The Boom of Social Media

Anastasia continues:

Social media helped us have the exposure I never would have thought we could have. We couldn't come this far without social media. Now, we are in every corner of the world.

Thanks to my daughter, we were early adopters on the Instagram platform. She saw it as an opportunity for the brand to expand through social media and build a special relationship with users. We took a grassroots approach by sending products to promising artists. Knowing that not everyone would use makeup the same way and that it would need to be customized from face to face, we were excited to showcase the diversity of what everyone was creating.

I remember the moment it hit me just how many more people we could reach. When we would travel to the salons at Nordstrom and spend time speaking with clients about the products, we would maybe reach one hundred people a day. It was all we could do with the time constraints. But when we posted those first images to Instagram, we were soon getting thousands of likes. A woman commented about how she wished she had Brow Wiz where she lived. I asked, "What's your address? I'll send you one." But she was in Pakistan! We had a fan all the way in Pakistan, and I then realized the kind of impact social media was going to allow us to have.

Now, it's a favorite part of my day seeing the creativity that comes from our followers, especially young people who aren't afraid to try new things and experiment. They are a constant source of inspiration.

Ahead of Her Time

Anastasia was always three steps ahead of everybody else.

Today, nearly everyone in the beauty industry takes inclusivity seriously, and it's amazing. When I started creating products two decades ago, nobody kept it top of mind. But for me, it was never even a question. When I launched the line in 2000, I wanted to have a color for every single client. We created products for every hair color, skin tone, and undertone so when a client walked into my salon, whether from Sweden, Hong Kong, or Nigeria, they could feel like the products were created for them.

We were among the first to post photos on our social media with men in our makeup. It seemed completely natural. Beauty doesn't have a gender. We support artistry, period. That support led us to become official sponsors of *RuPaul's Drag Race* before the show even became mainstream. The artistry of the drag queens was just incredible. Makeup is an art form and we are happy to support anyone who loves makeup and takes chances in expressing themselves artistically. We remained true to our core brand principles and our customers appreciated and embraced the authenticity and love we have for the craft as well as our stance on inclusivity.

Now my daughter, Claudia Soare, is doing some incredible work to continue that mission. She rallied consumers to encourage retailers to stock all fifty shades of our new liquid foundation and created waves with her Norvina Collection that is dedicated to artistic expression with bold color.

DR. BARBARA STURM

"I took my knowledge of orthopedics and put it into skin."

—DR. BARBARA STURM

Dr. Barbara Sturm is the German pioneering scientist behind the notorious "vampire facial,"[277] "blood creams," Sun Drops, Glow Drops, Hyaluronic Serum and Super Anti-Aging Serum that everyone is talking about. Dr. Sturm through her quality,

---

277 A "vampire facial" is a facial that consists of separating out the platelet-rich plasma and injecting it into the face to promote collagen production.

result-driven product and her celebrity-based clientele with Hailey Bieber, Gigi Hadid, Kim Kardashian West, Rosie Huntington-Whiteley, Gwyneth Paltrow, Kate Moss, and more raving about her noninvasive treatments, procedures and products, has built a cult following that expands all around the world but mainly across Europe and the US. Dr. Sturm has now been covered by *Elle, Style, Red, Vogue, Time, Gala, About Her* and many more due to her success and results.

Dr. Sturm's minimally invasive therapies with different focuses such as skin quality, skin structure, facial contours and skin firming complement each other perfectly.[278] Her mission with her Molecular Cosmetics brand is to make people *feel* and look more beautiful from the inside out and the outside in keeping their unique and natural beauty intact.

Applying Her Knowledge

Dr. Barbara Sturm told *Vogue*: [279]

> When I was four years old, I knew I wanted to become a doctor. My mom was a lab doctor and she took me to the hospital when I was a little girl. I

---

278 "Doctor And Team." 2019. *Dr-Barbara-Sturm.Com.* Accessed September 1 2019. https://www.dr-barbara-sturm.com/clinic/doctor-and-team/.

279 Ibid.

said, "Okay, that's what I want to do when I'm older!" I was born in a tiny village that was in the forest, so I was in the forest all day long looking for herbs. It's funny: I didn't plan to do anything with plants—it was just my interest.[280]

At first, I wanted to become a pediatrician. Then I had a daughter when I was twenty-three and I had to go into the pediatric clinic. I saw all these kids suffering, and I said, "No way can I do this!" It was too painful to picture my own daughter in these difficult situations. Since I was studying sports at the same time as medicine, I thought, "Okay, let's do orthopedics!" When I was done with my studies at school, I met a group of orthopedists and scientists and I helped pioneer a treatment against osteoarthritis. Essentially, we were taking blood and protein and tricking the cells into thinking there is a wound in the syringe that the cells have to help heal. All of a sudden, the cells produce these healing factors and we injected this healing factor into the joints.[281]

I was on my way to becoming a scientist when a doctor friend of mine told me, "This weekend I'm going

280 Nast, Condé. 2016. "*This Scientist And Beauty Guru's 9-To-5 Style Isn't Limited to A Lab Coat.*" *Vogue.* Accessed October 10 2019. https://www.vogue.com/article/barbara-sturm-cher-angela-bassett-kim-kardashian-west-beauty-scientist.

281 Ibid.

to learn how to inject lips!" This was fifteen years ago, and I was like, "I want to do that, too!" I learned how to inject wrinkles, lips, and I enjoyed the artistic nature of the work. And then I started injecting hyaluronic acid into wrinkles, but I thought, "That's not the treatment for me—I need to do something on the cellular level." I wanted to do something that really has a regenerative effect on the cells. I just transferred the knowledge from the orthopedics into the skin. And that's how it all started. [282]

I had seen great success in patients through a procedure that injects protein derived from a person's own blood into inflamed joints to reduce inflammation, mostly in cases of arthritis, to stimulate healing. So I thought: Why not apply this practice to the skin?[283]

Sliding into the Beauty Space

I only got into this space because I wanted to fix my own skin from dryness and blackheads, and I eventually did fix my own skin. I got facials every three weeks and tried every product on the market, but nothing worked. This is how I

---

282 Ibid.
283 "Dr. Barbara Sturm Has Bottled The Fountain Of Youth." 2019. *Forbes.Com*. Accessed October 10 2019. https://www.forbes.com/sites/addiewagenknecht/2018/05/08/dr-barbara-sturm-is-changing-how-we-age-or-dont/#68a726ef5eca.

ended up sliding into the beauty space. I came up with a product myself, the blood cream and then consequently a lot more products.

How did her cult favorite MC1 cream come about?

Dr. Barbara Sturm told *Time* magazine: [284]

> When I felt armed with enough information on how to create an effective line of products, I went to the lab and added proteins from my blood to a base that I developed and tested it out on myself. My skin woes were virtually resolved overnight.[285]

> Now I am happy with my skin. So that is all that matters. My goal is to make more people be happy with their skin. I can look at myself in the mirror and say, "Yes, I love how I look, and I love myself, and I feel comfortable leaving my house with no makeup on or no concealer on because I am confident that my skin is looking great." I think if you are self-conscious about your complexion it can disrupt your whole day and life.

---

284 Ibid.
285 Ibid.

Beauty is something that lies in your soul and helps with your own confidence. Having radiance and glowing skin you look beautiful. It's not about having perfectly smooth skin or no wrinkles. It's about the radiance in your skin. Worrying about your skin really disrupts your whole day and life.

Taking care of your skin is simple! You just have to have the best quality. You don't need to overload your skin with hundreds of products. [286]

Stay Away from Mis-Information

Dr. Barbara Sturm thinks technology is not doing its part for the beauty industry because it leads to a lot of lies and a digital marketing that is not conveying the correct information to consumers. "Big conglomerates are only focusing on a marketing game. They are very far removed from the consumer in comparison to a doctor that is able to meet with her clients on regular consultations and knows what they need and want."

I'm totally focused on effectiveness. If products don't work, I don't make them. If I am not obsessed about

286 Nast, Condé. 2016. "This Scientist And Beauty Guru'S 9-To-5 Style Isn'T Limited To A Lab Coat." *Vogue.* Accessed October 10 2019. https://www.vogue.com/article/barbara-sturm-cher-angela-bassett-kim-kardashian-west-beauty-scientist.

a product, I don't make it. If the products are going to irritate or inflame, I wouldn't use them, and I would not make them. I believe totally in my philosophy and the products are very much aligned with it too, and that is why they keep buying my products.

—DR. BARBARA STURM

The only way you can survive in this saturated market, with all the information available to the consumer, is by providing incomparable results; and she does. When I met Dr. Sturm she gave me a starter kit with half a dozen products, and I have to say that after only one month of using them I saw a visible difference in the way my skin looked. My personal favorites are Hyaluronic Acid and Glow Drops!

Dr. Barbara Sturm adds:

Now the beauty space has become about marketing and selling products and not about what clients want or need. It's all about how much more can I sell, instead of communicating with the consumer and asking them if they are actually happy with the product. Now it's more about a money-making machine than a need to give results.

There is too much coming out right now. Everyone thinks they need to be doing a skin care line these days. These are crazy times. I think there are so many skin care brands on the market. Now every celebrity is coming out with a skin care brand and it's just too hard to compete with all that is out there unless you are coming out with a super new and innovative scientific cutting-edge formula or technique. Other than this, we don't need more skin care lines, I think.

Plastic waste is also unethical to support, and companies should be more aware of this when they create their packaging.

Dr. Sturm projects a point where consumers will realize this tendency and start refusing to put poor quality products on their faces. They will stop because they want the truth, they want transparency about the ingredients in products, and they want honest and results-oriented brands. What you put on your skin is just as important as what you ingest because at the end of the day, the products you use topically seep into your dermis and blood stream in only about twenty minutes. Dr. Sturm thinks people should be willing to spend as much on what they put on their body as what they ingest.

Feel Beautiful in Your Own Skin

Dr. Sturm encourages all to be themselves, to *feel* beautiful in their own skin, and allow themselves to *feel* more beautiful by using honest and results-oriented products. Her products are meant to heal your skin mainly from inflammation and enhance your complexion as well as protecting you from any harm from the environment through her science-based formulas. There is nothing more beautiful than healthy bare skin in her opinion and her products help cultivate that, so you don't have to hide it with makeup. For this reason, her brand focuses on enhancing your natural beauty. Dr. Sturm only comes out with products she knows are effective and her marketing is built around results and science-backed information.

She agrees that there is an obvious call back to normality in terms of beauty in the industry, and this call stems from the excessive pull toward the very aggressive surgical and treatment-based procedures that completely alter one's looks.

We are tired of lies, photoshop, and harmful chemicals in our branded products. We want quality products based on science and medicine that are ethical and do no harm to the environment, animals, or the users themselves in primary or secondary effects. Products backed by science (her MC1 blood cream and her vampire facial) are scientific breakthroughs that are effective.

Including Everyone

Dr. Sturm tells *Forbes*, "I noticed a gap in the market to directly address the skin care needs of African-American women from prestige brands and I wanted to fix that."[287] During our talk, Dr. Sturm stressed how important being inclusive in her skin care products is to her and added, "We are actually the first skin care brand that came out with a line for people of darker skin tones. Now Fenty is coming out with one too, but we were the first ones."

Dr. Sturm also has a baby and children's line, which she invented for her own daughter, Pepper. In addition, she has also created a line for male skin care. She is really championing all aspects of inclusion, making all feel part of the conversation.

"I really do my best to educate people to help them heal their skin."

—DR. BARBARA STURM

She has taken it upon herself to teach people about skin care, ingredients, formulations, and applications of her products,

---

287 "Dr. Barbara Sturm Has Bottled the Fountain of Youth." 2019. *Forbes.Com*. Accessed October 10 2019. https://www.forbes.com/sites/addiewagenknecht/2018/05/08/dr-barbara-sturm-is-changing-how-we-age-or-dont/#68a726ef5eca.

and more through her Instagram. It is incredible to see genuine and honest information readily available from a renowned skin scientist. I have been watching her videos for almost a year now, and I have learned a lot.

PART IV

A TANGIBLE GIFT FROM THEM TO YOU

CHAPTER 10

BECOMING A SMARTER BEAUTY CONSUMER

———

We need to be so careful about social media and digital information overload. We now have so much readily accessible and digestible information at our fingertips.

The amount of time we spend on social media, how closely we follow influencers, and the hype around health, beauty, and wellness make us vulnerable to becoming compulsive consumers and buying anything that will make us *feel* better.

That's not to say that the beauty industry can't influence us in a healthy manner. It can if we protect ourselves and understand what we need to be looking out for. One of the best ways to protect yourself is to become a conscious consumer—one who buys and conforms to trends with intent and not as a bystander.

Being yourself and appreciating your beauty from within can be a difficult task for people who have not thought about beauty in this capacity. As I interviewed professionals for the book, some of them were willing to give me some recommendations for you in terms of how to be a smarter beauty consumer!

These recommendations vary widely—from what ingredients professionals think are worth investing in versus what to avoid, to routines and practices that you can begin implementing into your life to promote inside-out beauty.

SKIN COMES FIRST

As Dr. Barbara Sturm[288] says:

> I think if you are self-conscious about your complexion, it can disrupt your whole day and life. Beauty lies in your soul and helps with your own confidence. Having

---

288 Dr. Barbara Sturm is the founder and CEO of Dr. Barbara Sturm Molecular Cosmetics. She is a German aesthetics doctor, widely renowned for her anti-inflammatory philosophy and her non-surgical anti-aging skin treatments. Dr. Sturm translated science from her clinical research and orthopedic practice into the field of aesthetics and has been a success ever since.

radiance and glowing skin makes you look beautiful. An important thing to remember is that beautiful skin is not about having perfectly smooth skin or no wrinkles. It's about the radiance in your skin.

Now, I know this is a lot harder for some than for others. Skin conditions are treacherous, and for this we need to have patience and find the root cause of these flares from the inside out (lifestyle, food, allergies, stress, health). At times, the way our skin reacts is out of our control, but as long as our focus stays on having healthy skin through a healthy mind and body, all the other beauty enhancements are a plus.

Skin is the largest organ in the body and it often serves as a window to everything going on inside. Radiant skin usually signals a radiant inner beauty. Also, when we can work with a radiant clean canvas, we are free of having to use makeup to cover up our skin insecurities and onto utilizing makeup by choice.

When makeup is an option and not a necessity, we have an improved relationship with the beauty industry, as a way to adorn rather than as a medium to hide behind.

Routine for Prevention and Aging Beautifully

What should you be doing to make sure your skin is as radiant as can be for as long as can be?

Peter Thomas Roth Recommends: [289]

- Stay **protected** from the **sun!** Always apply sunscreen onto your face in the morning, before going outdoors—and don't forget about your chest, neck and hands, too! Wearing sunscreen on these areas is important because they easily show signs of sun damage and aging and are big giveaways of your actual age.

- It's also important to **reapply your sunscreen every couple of hours** since the effects can wear off after your initial application. Peter says the easiest way to stay protected from the sun throughout the day is to use his Instant Mineral Broad Spectrum SPF 45 Sunscreen, a translucent brush-on powder that's easy and sanitary to apply on the go.

- If you're not able to apply and reapply sunscreen, however, Peter recommends the following:

  - When **driving your car**, always wear **sunglasses and light gloves** to protect your delicate eye area and hands—while **UVB (burning)** rays don't penetrate your car window, **UVA (aging)** rays do. You can keep your gloves in the accessory pocket of your car door, so they're accessible. If wearing long sleeves and you don't have gloves, pull your **sleeves down to your fingers to**

---

289 Peter Thomas Roth is the CEO, founder, and formulator of Peter Thomas Roth Clinical Skin Care, is an influential segment leader in the beauty industry and continues to corner the clinical market as a groundbreaking, results-focused innovator. Today, Peter's comprehensive range of products are sold worldwide in over eighty countries, with Peter leading all research and development efforts at his state-of-the-art lab and manufacturing facility.

keep your hands protected. If not wearing long sleeves, keep a light throw blanket handy to drape over and protect your arms while driving. And, if you're in a **convertible, a baseball cap or hoodie** really works well.

- When walking around outside, try to walk on the shady side of the street to avoid direct sunlight.
- If you're not able to apply and reapply sunscreen, however, Peter recommends the following:
  - Apply a **Retinol** serum nightly to help **improve the look of fine lines, wrinkles, uneven skin tone, texture and radiance.** Peter uses a unique, pure and potent solution of Time-Released Microencapsulated Retinol in his Retinol Fusion PM Night Serum that delivers a gradual stream of non-irritating Retinol all night long while you sleep.

Dr. Ava Shamban Recommends: [290]

Dr. Shamban says, "Aging gracefully is very expensive if you don't do the right things. The way to approach skin care is by actually taking care of your skin, as obvious as that may sound. Using high quality skin care, staying away from the

---

290 Dr. Ava Shamban is the owner and director of two branded practices—AVA MD, her full-service Dermatology clinics in Santa Monica, Beverly Hills, and new concept SKINFIVE in West LA/Century City and Pacific Palisades. She is a renowned board-certified dermatologist, true skin visionary, clinician, author, anti-aging expert, prejuvenation proponent, and now co-host on The GIST Show.

sun and not trying to pretend to be young forever, meaning going to extreme measures. It's about respecting your skin"

- Use **sunscreen**! That should go without saying.
    - Make sure you are taking care of your chest as well.
- Get into **good life habits** and have a **holistic beauty** approach:
    - **Good nutrition**: we are not vessels for the microbiome (embodies your **beauty inside out)**. There is a huge **connection between gut health and skin.**
    - **Move** your body to get rid of toxic waste, which can sometimes come from stress and can cause breakouts.
    - Maintain better **sleeping** habits.
    - **Manage** your **stress levels.**
- Understand that what is important in life is your **health**, the people around you who **love** you, and having a **purpose.**
    - When you understand this and act on it, you will *feel* **beautiful** and be the **best version of yourself.**
- **Washing your face at night** is very important; not doing so is like not going to the bathroom all day!
    - All the pollutants in your skin from the day must be washed out.
- You should be using something in the **Retinae family** (it is the most effective and well-studied ingredient).
    - It increases **cell turnover**, reduces **pre-cancerous cells**, and evens out the **pigment** layer of your skin.

- People who use something in the Retinae family for an extended period have a drastically better complexion and better skin than people who don't.
- Using something in the **antioxidant** category is great.
  - An easy way to know if one is good is by looking at the list of ingredients on the back of the bottle. If it mentions antioxidants in the top part of the ingredients list, chances are the product has potent antioxidants (but again, this is just a quick way you can steer yourself in the right direction).
- Use products with **hyaluronic acid**, as it reduces the irritation of Retinol and is great for hydration.
- You should look for products that are **"clean,"** meaning that they are **safe** for the **skin.**
- You want to find products with **quality ingredients** and as **few ingredients** as possible (look in the back of the bottle).
- **Niacinamide** helps fight inflammation.

There is a consensus that we need to be disciplined with our skin care for it to age gracefully, and what stands between us and radiant aging skin is the sun. As much as we love to sunbathe, we should stay away from the sun and use protection as much as we can.

THE IRONY!

My parents have been telling me to put SPF on all my life.

I was always the little girl covered in sunscreen while all my friends looked bronzed and sun kissed. Of course, I always tried to scheme myself out of putting sunscreen on, so I could get tanned too. The problem was that I always got caught because I returned home from the beach looking like a lobster. And for me, that meant time out... as though the sunburn pain was not enough punishment.

My parents were extremely strict about sunscreen application and I always thought they were being so annoying.

You can imagine, living in Miami for some years while I was growing up, I experienced many of those painful sunburns together with the lectures from my parents.

Like everything in life, now I see why they would get so mad at me. Now, the irony is that I am a sunscreen fanatic. I fully understand the severe skin health repercussions from sunburns, not to mention the long-term aging effects. I probably have some waiting for me in the future after all those years of being the "lobster child" running around, but I hope I have redeemed myself at least a little. I now provide everyone with the 70+ SPF when we are out in the sun. My lesson has been learned. The more you protect yourself from the sun the healthier your skin will look down the line.

INGREDIENTS THAT ARE WORTH THE INVESTMENT

A huge question surrounding ingredients has been: When should I begin using Retinol or any other theoretically "anti-aging" ingredients?

Short answer, most ingredients are ageless and can benefit people of different ages for different reasons. It's more about your skin type.

I asked Peter Thomas Roth this question.

> Whether you're younger and just starting to see wrinkles or older with many wrinkles, the same anti-aging ingredients work on all ages and it's never too early to start working these ingredients into your routine. My anti-aging products also benefit younger customers because they can help preserve their youthful look while fighting off early signs of aging.

Peter Thomas Roth's List of Top Ingredients to Invest In:

- Retinol
- Vitamin C
- Collagen
- Hyaluronic Acid
- Peptides
- Neuropeptides
- AHAs (Glycolic Acid)
- Salicylic Acid
  - Peter says this ingredient is not only great for acne, which is what people tend to use Salicylic Acid for, but also great for helping to reduce the look of wrinkles!

Every company has their signature niche ingredient that gives their products their magical touch.

Peter's Signature Ingredients:

- Pumpkin Enzyme
- 24K Gold
- Cucumber Extract
- Hungarian Thermal Water
- Irish Moor Mud

Peter's motto is to combine potent natural ingredients like these with cutting-edge, scientific breakthrough ingredients that are safe and effective.

"When I'm sick, I want the chicken soup and the antibiotics!"

—PETER THOMAS ROTH

I'm going to eat my chicken soup, drink my tea with honey and get my Vitamin C, but I'm also going to take antibiotics, when needed and prescribed by a doctor. I love natural remedies side by side with antibiotics for maximum relief.

That's my motto and I apply the same philosophy to my skin care products. I add a lot of natural ingredients, but I also add a lot of safe scientific ingredients like peptides, neuropeptides and AHAs. We are in the twenty-first century and have this advanced technology and innovation to create amazing ingredients, so why not include those as well? For the most effective products and astonishing results, my theory is that whether ingredients are natural or clinical, it doesn't matter. You want to use what works best or a combination of both.

—PETER THOMAS ROTH

I stand by Peter's theory. This is also the belief of many other successful skin care creators like Dr. Sturm and Maria Calderon.[291]

EAT QUALITY INGREDIENTS AS WELL

Dr. Shamban recommends the following super foods for glowing skin:

- Avocados
- Almonds
- Beans
- Blueberries
- Eggs
- Green Tea
- Salmon
- Tomatoes
- Oranges
- Yellow Curry

Watching what we eat is undoubtedly one of the most important ways to ensure our beauty can shine from the inside

---

291 Maria Calderon is the CEO and founder of Kosmetai, founder of Institut Nahia, and founder of Juveskin, S.L. company, where she serves as Director General and is the Technical Director of PRODUCTOS BIORGANICOS, S.L. Maria is a chemical cosmetic pharmaceutical specialist and licensed expert in the evaluation of the security and information files of cosmetic products.

out. This way we are giving our body enough nutrients to fight inflammation and disease while maintaining our general health. Although you should think about taking in the right foods daily, with some space for some comfort foods of course, it is also a great idea to take supplements or nutricosmetics to make sure you are getting the proper amounts of nutrients and vitamins for a proper function of your body.

Fleur Phelipeau[292] cannot stress how essential it is to take the right nutricosmetics to reach our beauty goals. Being the leader in France for nutricosmetics, her goal is to enhance people's beauty and well-being with state-of-the-art micro-nutritionist ingredients, technologies, and formulas. Fleur says unfortunately we now live in a world where foods are processed, fruits and vegetables are grown in labs or depleted soil, and we leave food in refrigerators for far too long, which exhausts it from all of its vital nutrients. Therefore, we do not have enough nutrients in what we eat to ensure optimal bodily functions and inner harmony with one's physical and mental health.

Fleur explains:

---

292 Fleur Phelipeau is the CEO and Founder of D-LAB Nutricosmetics, Birdie Nutrition, and Claude Aphrodisiacs. She has surrounded herself with doctors from Vichy Célestins ever since she was a little girl, which played a huge role in her innate affinity for hyper-nutrition beauty from within. Nutricosmetics are Fleur's passion; she has been working with them for over fifteen years.

Outer beauty is inherently connected with how our body is doing inside. When we start understanding the symbiotic relationship with everything in our body, we begin to realize where we should be investing more in nutricosmetic formulas that contain micronutrients such as vitamins, minerals, and good bacteria that will satisfy the needs of our body's cells and functions in order to give us the long-term boost, vitality, and radiance we are all looking for in topical products.

Nutricosmetic formulas can get our body to tackle beauty from the root in order for all other beauty routines on top of this one to be more effective. The wear and tear of life such as stress, fatigue, and this "go, go, go" lifestyle we all live in cause hormonal imbalances and weakened immune and nervous systems. This is yet another factor that hinders our normal bodily functions.

Results-proven nutricosmetics such as ours, at D-LAB Nutricosmetics, have been formulated in such a way so as to ensure each dose contains the correct amount of active ingredients needed to obtain and protect that equilibrium between our mind and body. Eventually, I believe people will come to recognize that nutricosmetics is a "must" and not a "should" in everyone's beauty routine with the goal of approaching beauty with a more holistic philosophy.

Nutricosmetics are indeed not a replacement of a healthy diet. They should be implemented in addition to one. Fleur recommends looking into nutricosmetics if you have not before because they guarantee your body the adequate amount of nutrients it needs, which is unattainable due to the food conditions of today, to perform at our best and *feel* our best every day, championing your beauty from within.

TWELVE-STEP ROUTINE NOT NEEDED!

With so many YouTube and IGTV skin care tutorials out there where they use a million skin care products at a time, we are starting to think that a "proper" skin care routine should have twelve or more steps. This is not necessarily true. If twelve steps work for you and make you *feel* beautiful, by all means do it! But if you are looking for potency and effectiveness or you don't have a huge budget to spend on beauty products, you don't need such a long routine to see magnificent results.

Below is my routine in case you want an example. I have been doing this routine for about a year now, and I have never had better skin than I do now. I pair my routine with my face mask sessions, which I personally find the most therapeutic "me-time" moments of the day.

Quality Steps I take:

Morning Routine

1. Double Cleanse
2. Essence
3. Hyaluronic acid
4. Moisturizer with SPF 40

Night Routine

1. Double Cleanse (same as morning)
2. Essence (same as morning)
3. Retinol Serum
4. Face oil (Rose hip or Noni)

**This routine works for me but does not mean it will work for everyone's skin type. I am twenty-two years old, and I have sensitive, combination, and fair skin.[293]

** The brands of the products I use are not marked as I am still doing trial periods on the ones that work best on my skin.

---

293 Skin spectrum: dry, combination, oily skin.

I am no dermatologist or doctor, but I can assure you that with these products and investing in a four-step morning and night routine, you can get your skin very far. You don't need to buy twelve products, nor do you need to be up on all the beauty trends because that only confuses your skin.

The Greater China Vice President of one of the world's leading beauty multinational companies told me her beauty routine and I want to share it with you. This way you also have an example of a skin routine for a middle-aged individual.

The Greater China Vice President multinational beauty company's skin care routine:[294]

Morning Routine
1. Double Cleanse with two different face washes
2. Lotion
3. Serum
4. Moisturizer
5. UV protector

Night Routine
1. Double Cleanse with two different face washes
2. Watery Lotion
3. Eye Cream

---

294 This industry professional wishes to keep personal and company information anonymous.

4. Repair Serum
5. Moisturizer
6. Sheet Mask

We always wonder about the order in which we should apply different steps of our routine; these two routines are examples of the best order in terms of maximum absorption. However, if you already have a routine that works for you, and you want to make sure you are doing the steps in the right order, make sure you apply products from the lightest viscosity to the heaviest viscosity, so the molecules can penetrate the layers of skin they are engineered to. In other words, the most liquid to the oiliest does the trick!

Peter and Dr. Shamban both believe that using many skin care products inconsistently may cause an adverse effect on your skin. The mix of various active ingredients can produce unwanted results, inflammation, or other side effects. Furthermore, they think using too many products can inhibit you from learning what works on your skin and what doesn't.

Another thing to keep in mind is that your skin does not start giving you results until the third or fourth week of using a product. Hence, we should keep our skin care routines consistent and try to have quality products that will give us those results that we want.

DON'T BE A VICTIM OF *GREENWASHING*!

Arden Martin[295] recommends a handful of clean brands in order to avoid being a victim of Greenwashing.

Arden Martin's Recommendations:

Any of the brands in the Counter Act Coalition,[296] bringing safe cosmetics to consumers because to be provided with safe cosmetics is our right.

- Beautycounter
- Annmarie Gianni Skin Care
- Biossance
- Côte
- Credo
- Follain
- Goddess Garden
- Innersense Organic Beauty
- Josie Maran
- May Lindstrom
- OSEA

---

295 Arden Martin is a teacher of Vedic Meditation and co-founder of The Spring Meditation Studio in New York City. She cares deeply about bringing more transparency to the US personal care industry and works with Beautycounter to educate people about what "clean beauty" really means.

296 Counter Act Coalition is a collective of more than twenty clean, high-performance beauty brands and its debut in Washington, DC in 2017, led by Beautycounter founder and CEO Gregg Renfrew.

- Peet Rivko
- Primal Pit Paste
- Rahua Hair Care
- RMS beauty
- Seventh Generation
- Silk Therapeutics
- SkinOwl
- S.W. Basics
- Tenoverten
- The Detox Market
- Vapour Organic Beauty

Arden's Top Picks:

- Beautycounter (All clean cosmetics)
- RMS beauty (Clean makeup)

TOXIC "NESS" AND CLEAN "NESS"

Although it is difficult for us to know if an ingredient is toxic or not, these websites/applications are mentioned in chapter 5 and can be helpful in pointing out whether a product is safe or not.

Websites/Apps to Find Out if a Product Is Clean:

- Think Dirty

- GoodGuide
- CosmeEthics
- EWG Skin Deep
- Detox Me
- Dirty Dozen

Stay Away From:[297]

1. **Carbon Black:** used in some mascaras and is known to be a carcinogen.

2. **Formaldehyde:** some Keratin products contain this, and it is a well-known carcinogen.

3. **Mercury:** potent neurotoxin. A lot of people take care of the amount of mercury intake with fish, but makeup has it too.

Nneka also says we should not only be aware of the dermal and oral toxicity of a product, but also the inhalant toxicity.[298] For example, formaldehyde excretes some of its main toxicity from the residue left in the air that one inhales as they are having their hair straightened, and it is going straight into your lungs and bloodstream.[299] Keep in mind, however, that just because

---

297 "Why Are There Still Toxic Ingredients In Beauty Products? | Goop." 2019. *Goop.* Accessed October 6 2019. https://goop.com/beauty-closet-podcast/why-are-there-still-toxic-ingredients-in-beauty-products/.

298 Ibid.

299 Ibid.

a product says, "formaldehyde-free," for example, that does not mean there is not another ingredient in the product that has the same effect on your health as formaldehyde.[300] Try to look at the whole ingredient list and not just at targeted words.

Another example is when products say, "paraben free."[301] When we see that, we should not immediately presume that this product is safe to use because the product might be using another preservative that is arguably worse.

Just think, *"How are they making sure this product has a shelf life?"* and read the ingredients on the back of the product. The easiest thing to do is to use those apps I have mentioned above to get a clear idea on how safe a product is.

Tyle Mahoney's Recommendations:

Tyle Mahoney[302] also recommends being cautious with what we put in our hair when coloring it. The ingredients you put

---

300 Ibid.

301 Parabens are a type of preservative, first introduced in the 1950s. They're used to prolong shelf life in many health and beauty products by preventing the growth of mold and bacteria within them.

302 Tyle Mahoney is an expert colorist with more than fifteen years of experience at MèCHE salon. Clients depend on him not only for his skill when it comes to creating the perfect color, but also for his ability to make his creations lastlast. Considering lifestyle as well as the elements, Tyle tailors his methods to ensure fade-resistant color and shine. He works hand in hand with Tracey Cunningham.

on your hair are not so frequently looked at and they should be, he says.

Be conscious of all the hair products you use!

- Ingredients: make sure they are **clean products.**
- Environment: use **products** that will work right with your hair in terms of the **climate** you are in.
- **Hair type:** as much as it is important to use skin care for your skin type, it is equally as important to use hair products that work well for your hair.
  - For example, if you have **fine hair,** you won't want to use conditioner, more like a spray leave-in conditioner.
- Olaplex is the brand to use.
  - It is a revolutionary formula and no product performs like it (according to Tyle).

QUALITY = $$$?

We all want the best treatments, the best quality ingredients, the best serums, the best creams, the best, best, best. All these "bests," but that means $$$.

Thankfully this is a myth. Some products are absolutely magical but are not too expensive at all.

We Can Do Two Things:

1. We can use very simple and less expensive ingredients (honey, aloe vera, rosehip oil, etc..) and more affordable products and simple effective skin routines to look our best. It takes more research but now it is much more affordable if $$$ concerns us.

2. You don't need to have a twelve-step beauty routine. You-can have a three step one and it can benefit your skin just as much if you are using good quality ingredients. While speaking to all of these professionals, I realized many of the best ingredients can be found in foods in your kitchen.

Maria Calderon told me before you pay for an expensive yet not "well-known" product, know that the high price does not always mean quality. We need to note that texturing ingredients in the cosmetic world can be just as expensive as the active ingredients of the product you are buying. For this reason, if you are buying a product that has a very special texture, think about the price and be conscious about the fact that you may be paying that amount for that interesting texture and not the actual quality of the ingredients. I personally thought this was very interesting, and I now always use the "try me" at the stores in order to keep an eye out. Keep in mind, however, if the brand is of very high quality, it is very possible that they have great quality ingredients alongside equally high-quality texturing ones. This is more something to keep an eye out for in the mid-range product, so you can gauge the price versus the quality.

I have been using home remedies as face masks, which have worked wonders. I use four quality products on my face every morning.

Face Masks Regularly I Use:

1. **"Honey-Head":** One teaspoon of Manuka Honey (or any raw honey) & 3 drops of Lemon.
   a. This combo has a powerful effect on your skin with its antibacterial and exfoliating properties. Manuka is good for improving the PH level of your skin and fading scarring and inflammation from acne. The lemon drops will give you a natural Vitamin C kick, reducing free radical damage caused by UV radiation.
   b. I leave it for about ten to fifteen minutes and do it two to three times a week.
   c. Your skin will look and *feel* radiant after this!
2. **Extra Virgin Olive Oil and Brown Sugar:** Two teaspoons of extra virgin olive oil and one teaspoon of brown sugar.
   a. Great natural exfoliant and moisturizer. The olive oil is a great antioxidant for your face and can help with signs of aging. The brown sugar acts as a gentle exfoliant, scrubbing the dead skin cells away.

b. I do this two to three times a week (not on the same days as "Honey-head").

3. **Aloe Vera:** Rub some fresh aloe from the leaf you can buy in the grocery store.
   a. Aloe is great for many things. Amongst them are natural hydration, cooling, alleviating irritation and inflammation, and acting as a natural antimicrobial.
   b. I do this as much as I can!

4. **"Yogurt-Face":** Two to three teaspoons of Greek Yogurt lathered generously on your face and neck. (This was taught to me by my sixty-year-old Russian host mother when I lived in St. Petersburg. Her skin was always vibrant and she was convinced this was the reason why.)
   a. Yogurt can help with the diminishing of wrinkles and fine lines as well as with the tightening of pores to give your face a little lift when your skin looks dull.
   b. I do this whenever I remember!

5. **Korean Sheet Masks:** This is recent and I use them before doing my makeup for an event or something special.
   a. These have different benefits depending on which ones you use.

AYURVEDIC BEAUTY ROUTINES

Roya Pourshalchi[303] gives us some of her favorite and easy to incorporate Ayurvedic traditions[304] to give us a more holistic approach to beauty.

Five Tips for Vitality & Longevity:

1. **Rising and Sleeping:** The number one rule of Ayurveda is regularity, so a simple step you can take toward natural beauty is to rise and sleep with the sun.
   a. This regulates your internal clock and your internal bodily functions.

2. **Drinking a cup of copper infused water:** Every morning fifteen minutes before breakfast on an empty stomach. You let water sit in a copper cup overnight for roughly eight hours and drink it in the morning.
   a. It is a natural antimicrobial that helps with circulation and collagen production in your body to have nice bones, skin, and nails. It also levels out the PH in the body and helps eliminate waste properly to

---

303 Roya Pourshalchi is a dedicated yoga teacher, Ayurveda consultant at Kilona Shop, and Marma bodywork therapist. Roya currently sees clients privately and hosts group classes and workshops in New York City. She is Yoga Alliance RYT-200 certified, trained in 100 HR Ayurveda Foundations and 100 HR Marma Therapy.

304 Ayurveda is a system of Indian traditional medicine (the sister science of yoga) based on the five elements in the world that are also within us: ether, air, water, fire and earth.

keep a healthy gut, where the root of most health issues begins.

3. **Dry brushing:** Great especially during the warmer seasons.

   a. This helps activate lymphatic drainage, exfoliate dead skin, and bring the energy to the center of your body by always brushing toward your heart.

4. **Tongue scrape:** Our body detoxes while we sleep. First thing in the morning, scrape your tongue seven to fourteen times downward to remove the toxicity that's accumulated over night. Your tongue is a window to all your organs, so when you scrape, you are waking up the digestive system for the day by doing this.

   a. When you sleep at night your body produces a residue on your tongue that is often odor causing bacteria that is not beneficial to keep in your mouth.

5. **Abhyanga massage (Body oil massage):** Massage yourself with oil each day (use sesame oil in the cold months and coconut oil in the warmer months). Apply the oil with long strokes on the bones and circles on the joints. Spend time massaging your belly clockwise to help with digestion. Let this sit for twenty minutes and then rinse off in the shower. Wash only the hairy areas of your body since the oil is naturally antimicrobial.

   a. You will *feel* your body relax. It will promote deeper sleep while nourishing the nervous system, skin and joints. In this day and age, we spend so much time in our mind and it's so important to get that energy back into our physical form.

CLEAR THROUGH THE NOISE

With social media becoming a constant digital marketing platform for products, treatments, ingredients, and beauty trends, transparency and efficacy are becoming more blurred. It is now becoming a lot harder to be an informed and conscious consumer.

It is also harder to become an expert on knowing exactly what ingredient is safe and the best for each of us to use without being lured by marketing and trends. We would all need to be chemists and dermatologists, or companies would have to be completely transparent about the ingredients they put in their products for us to be fully aware individuals.

Since that is not going to happen anytime soon, hopefully these key questions will at least steer you in the right direction toward becoming a better beauty consumer.

Olga Lorencin[305] Recommends to Ask Yourself the Following before You Buy:

- *Who made the product?*
- *Who is behind this brand?*
- *Do they have experience in the field?*
- *Are they passionate about skin care? Or is this just a business plan?*
- *Is this just another "me too" or "copy-cat" product?*
- *Is this a clinical brand?*

Ultimately, when buying skin care, you should be able to have a good and reasonable explanation as to why you are buying that brand. Remember, "Your skin doesn't need that much!" says Olga. She truly believes we should be investing our money in clinical or medical skin care for maximum results.

Your skin needs few products, but the right products. Since it is hard to figure out if some ingredients or formulations actually work for your skin, your safest bet is to base your choice of purchase on the mastermind behind the brand and formulation. It is almost impossible even for chemists and professionals to know what is in proprietary formulas nor

---

305 Olga Lorencin is the owner of Olga Lorencin Skin Care Clinic and CEO and founder for Olga Lorencin Skin Care. She is a top-tier esthetician and skin care guru and has spent more than twenty years in the treatment room studying ingredients. Olga is affectionately referred to as "The Acid Queen."

how they will react on their skin unless they try them on. So, it is better to stick to companies that give you good answers to the questions above and ones that you trust.

WE CARE ABOUT SUSTAINABILITY AND EFFICIENCY

Olga says sustainability is key, but biodegradable or recyclable packaging is not enough. For Olga, the most sustainable philosophy in skin care is not to make one. If there is no burning passion for making skin care or cutting-edge formula that will revolutionize the market, don't make another skin care line. "We don't need to have 30,000 brands of hyaluronic acids with sustainable bottles," she says.

For makeup, it is different because the more choices we have, the more included and beautiful we will all feel. But skin care can do with less waste, something Dr. Sturm mentioned as well.

Both Olga and Dr. Sturm agree that maybe we need some sort of qualification or verification to regulate the skin care market. Olga believes the regulation would be best if brands were required to have credible R&D, lab, researchers, dermatological, or cosmetic formulation experience in the past to be able to produce and sell products. Too many people are coming out with skin care lines but are simply not qualified to do so.

Olga gave an example.

> Imagine if my fourteen-year-old daughter came and told me, "Mom I want to make a new serum." If gave her a chemist, she could perfectly make one with the chemist and take it out to market in a few months. There is absolutely no regulation nor certifications needed. Now people just put skin care out on the market and let it sell with marketing stories.
>
> When are we going to figure it out?
>
> When will we learn to resist compulsory consumption and sophisticated marketing?

How much will we, as consumers, be willing to dig before we buy a product or buy into a brand? Olga says, "This is the biggest question that will penetrate every market, not only beauty."

For now, usually the people who have problematic skin dig deeper into skin care brands and products to find a correct solution to their conditions, but shouldn't we all?

Eventually, I believe people will get wiser and ask: "Why you? Why this formula? Why these ingredients? How much experience do you have?" That is the bottom line.

Things to remember:

- Don't be a hackable consumer. Be a conscious one.
- Focus on having healthy skin and what you put on it. Your skin reflects what is going on internally.
- Learn to celebrate your features. You may want to enhance yourself, but don't change yourself to the standards and trends.
- Foster self-confidence, self-love, and a healthy perspective.
- Your authenticity makes you beautiful.

Spend less investing in the way a product makes you look and invest more in the way a product makes you **feel.**

CHAPTER 11

SUCCEED IN YOUR BEAUTY BUSINESS

———

"Beauty is not shallow. Beauty is serious business. Your appearance speaks before you do and should say all that matters. Whether its leading the boardroom, or simply going through the day, we all do better Beauty-fully empowered."

—YUSEFF SMYTH, NEW YORK CITY

HAIRDRESSER AND IMAGE MAKER[306]

———

306 "Yuseff Smyth, Downtown NY Image-Maker." 2019. *The Leading Salons of The World.* Accessed October 2 2019. https://www.leadingsalons.com/en/beauty-expert/7/yuseff_smyth_downtown_ny_image-maker.

Beauty marketers, business owners, entrepreneurs, innovators, intrapreneurs, etc... this is for you.

Successful and relevant beauty businesses respect who you are as a person and acknowledge you as inherently special. These companies help you accentuate your Signature Features, pushing inner beauty to the surface.

The beauty industry has gone through some drastic shifts for the better, becoming more representative of the society we live in today, but we still have a long way to go. As I interviewed top professionals in the industry, I asked for some tips that they could give to up-and-coming professionals in the industry or ones who are thinking about joining it.

A LIFE DEDICATED TO YOUR PASSION

Known as the "Eyebrow Queen," Anastasia Soare[307] is one of the most successful self-made women in the beauty industry. From building a one-woman business from the ground up to working with the likes of Michelle Obama, Kris Jenner,

---

307 Anastasia Soare is the founder, CEO, and driving force behind Anastasia Beverly Hills—one of the fastest-growing brands in the beauty industry. In 1990, she introduced a new brow shaping technique to clients—later patented as the Golden Ratio Eyebrow Shaping Method—that has gone on to become a modern beauty essential. Anastasia is a beauty pioneer and powerhouse.

Oprah Winfrey, and many, many more, Anastasia has learned to be humble.

"Oprah Winfrey has been a client of mine since 1998. I've learned so much from her. I consider her a mentor. This is a woman who is the humblest, the smartest, the most giving. What I've learned from her over the years is that if you want to be successful, you can't do anything better than just working extremely hard."

—ANASTASIA SOARE

According to Anastasia, that is the most important thing she has learned from all these years in the business.

Anastasia humbly says:

> I owe everything to everyone. To every customer, every friend, every single person who supported me from day one. I would not be the same Anastasia I was thirty years ago without them. Yes, I built this incredible business, and I'm very proud. But I will not stop doing what I did three decades ago—work as hard as my first day every day.

It's amazing to speak with Anastasia because you can feel just how much she cares about her clients. Every single thing she has ever done while building her brand, Anastasia Beverly Hills, was for them.

BLURRED LINES: WORK AND PERSONAL LIFE

Anastasia continues:

> My work is my life. If you can equate the two, you'll enjoy every moment. I enjoy attending conferences, speaking at panels, working on my products, reading comments on social media and providing responses—everything. I like to learn constantly from my followers, from my consumers, and I get to do it every day. I'll never stop. I think I actually need the work, and that without it, I would be like a plant without sunlight. It gives me energy. It gives me life.

Jeanne Chavez says:[308]

> I always tell everyone who asks me how I do it: "Do your homework."

---

308 Jeanne Chavez is the President and co-founder of the beauty brands, Smith & Cult, and the co-founder of Hard Candy. She has had a decades-long career in beauty, starting off at Orlane Institute to luxury brand La Prairie before ending up at her current position.

Just because you love wearing makeup, and you love shopping for beauty products, for me, it really isn't enough for you to go out and create your own brand. Find out what you want to do, and then look at the next five years because you're going to be working really hard. I am always working. For me, my personal life and my work life are the same thing.

You need to love it so much, that even in your off-time, you are thinking of new ideas. Even if it's in your head. My "off-time" is where I spend a lot of time thinking about what's next. For me there are blurred lines between my personal life and my professional life.

I'll give you a really straightforward example. My vacations for many years were going places where I could either buy innovative beauty products, look at trends that I thought were amazing, or could experience a new way people perceived beauty. I would pick places where I knew I would find this when thinking of my vacation plans. My downtime is still my work time. Because everything I do has to inspire me to work. I really love to give that advice because I think if you can make that work, it's so rewarding.

BUT REALLY, DO YOUR HOMEWORK

Maybe we really should consider doing our homework. All these superstar professionals keep emphasizing it.

Anastasia Soare says, "Do your homework. Become the best in what you want to do."

> I wanted to do eyebrows and I wanted to become the best at doing eyebrows. Learn, be humble, be alert, see how everybody else does it and learn it in whatever way you have to do. Stop complaining. It's a lot of work. You have to love it. And that's the most important. You have to love it because it's so difficult that if you don't love it, you will give up. You need to love what you do; this is the most important thing.

Éstee Lauder herself said, "I didn't get there by wishing for it or hoping for it, but by working for it." [309]

As Anastasia Soare also states:

> You need to practice a minimum of 10,000 dedicated hours to that craft. There is no such thing as fast

---

309 "Huffpost Is Now A Part Of Verizon Media." 2019. *Huffpost.Com.* Accessed November 7 2019. https://www.huffpost.com/entry/ estee-lauder-quotes-beauty-business_n_3506334.

success. You cannot take the elevator. You have got to take the steps... I promise you it's possible. I came to the US without speaking English. So, you have an advantage. If I was able to do it, you could do it too. Everybody can do what I did. You just need to believe in yourself.

Look in the mirror every morning and say: "Anastasia did it. I can do it too."

CONSUMER-CENTRIC BEAUTY

Being consumer-centric is one of, if not the most important, asset of your company, brand, or service in the beauty industry.

Understand Your Consumer
Listen to Your Consumer

"I think the fundamental thing is to know the consumer: their values, their tastes, what moves them, their interests ... And then, adapt and communicate to this group, considering the parameters analyzed. I also find it interesting to incorporate millennials into the discussion and decision-making forums of large beauty companies (and in general, of any other type)."

—YOLANDA SACRISTÁN

Anastasia Soare agrees.

> It is critical that brands really listen to their con-
> sumers. I wake up every single morning and I want
> to know what's going through the mind of the ABH
> community. I want to know if they love a product,
> how they're using it, and what else they might need.
> I believe in order to create something of value, a
> company must remain committed to quality and
> fulfill a specific niche. When I created the first brow
> products, I was closing a gap in the market. And to
> expect people to invite me and my products into
> their daily routines requires a certain trust that as a
> brand we are going to deliver the best. I'll always give
> my best to ensure my clients feel their most beautiful.

BEAUTY BRANDING

Having a Clear Brand DNA

Clémence von Mueffling[310] once heard some of the best advice
on branding from a woman who worked at the Boston Consulting Group in beauty industry cases. The BCG Consultant

---

310 Clémence von Mueffling is the Founder and Editor of Beauty and
Well-Being (BWB), which brings a fresh aesthetic to the beauty
and well-being media. She is also the author of *Ageless Beauty the
French Way*, a luxurious, entertaining, unparalleled guide to every
French beauty secret for all women.

said that brands need a very clear idea of what they want to, and a very strong brand identity. It needs to be so clear that you should be able to draw a caricature of your brand. If you cannot describe your brand in a single sentence, it is not clear enough for the public. The brand is the soul of a beauty business. It must be consistent through and through.

Klara Chrzuszcz[311] emphasized the importance of not only having a clear DNA but also revisiting it when making business decisions and making sure those choices are being made with your consumers in mind. Klara said, "First you have to make a decision if you're going to target a small audience or mass produce. Some brands want their product to target all ages and all societies in the world while others are choosing a much more specific demographic." It is important to understand what consumer your branding is attracting and stay consistent with it.

A great example of this is Dr. Shamban.[312] She found herself in a situation where she had to assess the future of

---

311 Klara Chrzuszcz is a Medical Skin care Aesthetician, Clinical Skin care Expert, and the owner of Klara Beauty Lab. Klara is an educator in Europe for neurotoxin application as well as dermal fillers for the face and body, and she travels to teach on a yearly basis. Her approach involves delving into clients' lifestyles, diets, stress levels, etc. which, allows her to create a one-of-a-kind experience.

312 Dr. Ava Shamban is the owner and director of two branded practices—AVA MD, her full-service Dermatology clinics in Santa Monica, Beverly Hills, and new concept SKINFIVE in West LA/Century City and Pacific Palisades. She is a renowned board-certified dermatologist, true skin visionary, clinician, author, anti-aging expert, prejuvenation proponent, and now co-host on The GIST Show.

her brand values and whether she wanted to join a skin care brand that was doing very well yet had a different philosophy than hers. Dr. Shamban was offered work with Guthy Renker;[313] however, Dr. Shamban did not accept their proposal as she didn't think that her brand's DNA fit correctly with Guthy Renker's clients and sales model. "For me, my expansion was more focused on patient care and upscale products," Dr. Shamban notes. Now she has two SKINFIVE locations and two AVA MD locations in Los Angeles. She says, "I care more about the quality and the use of technology to achieve the highest results, rather than to scale thoughtlessly."

"In general, to have a successful brand or idea come along, you need to have ethics and you need to have a passion that is consistent with who you are as a person."

—DR. AVA SHAMBAN

How to Define Your Brand?

Questions to ask yourself proposed by a large conglomerate head that wished to remain anonymous:

---

313 Guthy Renker is one of the world's largest and most respected direct marketing companies. Since 1988, Guthy Renker has discovered and developed dozens of well-loved, high quality consumer products in the beauty, skin care, entertainment and wellness categories.

1. What does your brand believe in?
2. What is your mission?
3. What is your universe?
4. What will make consumers dream beyond the product?

Clear Philosophy

Peter Thomas Roth[314] maintains his momentum and credibility with his brand and skin care lines because every product he launches, whether it be a cleanser, toner, moisturizer, night cream or mask, "is a hero on its own." It can be bought and used by itself. By this he means his products can be used alone, in combinations with other Peter Thomas Roth products, or in combination with any other brand's products. He supports this idea because when you envision a woman showing you her bathroom cabinet or her skin care regimen nowadays, there are about twenty different brands. He feels this trend has started happening over the past twenty-five years and has been part of his brand's success. In the past, a woman would turn over her bag and you would see all one line or at least all one brand—all Clinique, all Estée Lauder, Clarins—but now this has changed.

---

314 Peter Thomas Roth is the CEO, founder, and formulator of Peter Thomas Roth Clinical Skin Care, is an influential segment leader in the beauty industry and continues to corner the clinical market as a groundbreaking, results-focused innovator. Today, Peter's comprehensive range of products are sold worldwide in over eighty countries, with Peter leading all research and development efforts at his state-of-the-art lab and manufacturing facility.

Peter recommends making products that can be integrated into a routine someone already has. He adds, "My skin care line has a multitude of products for every skin type and concern, so a consumer can easily find what they need for their personal routine. I never know whether someone will get just one of my products or a full cabinet, so I work with my chemists in my state-of-the-art lab and manufacturing facility to ensure every single product is truly breakthrough and effective. This way, no matter what a consumer chooses—either one product or an entire regimen of mine—they can trust it's going to deliver results."

Not all brands have this philosophy. Klara Chrzuszcz explained that she believes some brands should be purchased as a complementary regimen because their products and formulations work symbiotically with each other.

Both philosophies work very well, giving the consumer the option to choose between what they stand behind most. You need to be real and make sure whichever of the two you pick aligns most with your brand, is true for your products, and you confidently communicate it. That will help you maintain consumer loyalty.

Maria Calderon[315] champions total transparency with the effectiveness of products and the results they bring. She is a true believer of before and after photos for any product in the industry.

In the end, if all brands are the best in one certain product or type of product, all brands win because it is hard to remain loyal to a single brand with all the innovation and creativity surging through the industry. For your brand to succeed, you need to make certain you are offering a product that is the best at expressing a certain feeling, look, or emotion.

Why does your brand work?

Shadoh Punnapuzha:[316] "I believe my brand works because I am focused on the holistic, identity, cultural, and representational part of beauty. This is the way I stay true to myself and the brand and stay authentic and relevant."

---

315 Maria Calderon is the CEO and founder of Kosmetai, founder of Institut Nahia, and founder of Juveskin, S.L. company, where she serves as Director General and is the Technical Director of PRODUCTOS BIORGANICOS, S.L. Maria is a chemical cosmetic pharmaceutical specialist and licensed expert in the evaluation of the security and information files of cosmetic products.

316 Shadoh Punnapuzha is the Founder of Taïla Skincare. She is proving that when you combine the power of Ayurveda and science, you get divine results. After years of working at a PE firm in NYC and going through a burnout, Shadoh found her path to a healthy life and a healthy skin through Ayurveda.

Dr. Alouie:[317] "First of all, your product should have something new and convincing about it so the consumer trusts it. Secondly, the underlying message should be a message of confidence and empowerment."

Stephanie Peterson:[318] "Doing tutorials of how you use my products, and their manufacturing process gives my consumers a sense of the integrity and transparency I ensure in my marketing, ingredients and products. Another important component of success is having an open line of communication with your consumers. Lastly, I just do it because I love it and fully believe in it."

Dr. Sturm:[319]

> I think my brand works because I am totally focused
> on effectiveness; if a product doesn't work, I don't

317 Dr. Jouhayna Alouie is a well-known esthetician in Beirut, Paris, and Riyadh, who has been working in the field since the mid-seventies. She specializes in corrective work, permanent makeup, and enhancement facial treatments. In the past, she has worked closely with Miss France and many Arab celebrities.

318 Stephanie Peterson is a model and the founder of Smoothie Beauty, a clean and organic skin care line that is truly fresh without any toxic chemicals, additives, or preservatives, and creator of The Global Beauty blog. She has modeled in 15+ countries, with the likes of Clinique, Mary Kay and Pandora, among others.

319 Dr. Barbara Sturm is the founder and CEO of Dr. Barbara Sturm Molecular Cosmetics. She is a German aesthetics doctor, widely renowned for her anti-inflammatory philosophy and her non-surgical anti-aging skin treatments. Dr. Sturm translated science from her clinical research and orthopedic practice into the field of aesthetics and has been a success ever since.

make it or sell it. If I am not obsessed about a product, I don't make it. If a product irritates or inflames, I would not use it, so I would not make it. I believe totally in our philosophy and I think it is obvious that I really care about results and that is why my clients keep buying my products.

Peter Thomas Roth:

I put all my ingredients on the front of my products in big font. I was the pioneer of this. I just put it out there because I want my customers to know everything in my products and their percentage. I believe my brand works because my products use the most effective ingredients at the maximum strength possible. I include the percentage of active ingredients on all my products, so you know what you're getting, and you know it delivers astonishing results! I'm all about transparency.

Klara Chrzuszcz:

I don't concern myself with competitors. I do what I love and make sure I am always giving it my all for my clients and myself. If you consistently provide your clients with quality service and go above and beyond for them, they will be loyal to you. For this reason, I am able to build my clientele with word of mouth and trust. Having passion for my career, staying true and honest to what I believe, and showing my clients that their happiness and satisfaction is in the forefront of everything I do is how I continue to be successful.

COMMUNICATING YOUR STORY
TO DIFFERENT MARKETS

Brands can learn to tell the stories of many individuals from different cultures, in ways so individuals can feel identified in a unique way with a certain name.

Franck Moison[320] explains the importance of a clear story and finding a way to resonate with the audience. As the Head of Greater China beauty business at a leading multinational corporation[321] says, "If the brand wants to operate successfully in the Asian market, they need to be in Asia. It doesn't matter how successful a brand was in the US or Europe. You need to re-interpret the brand essence with cultural relevance and resonance."

---

320 Franck Moison is the former Chief Operating Officer and Vice Chairman of Colgate-Palmolive. He is an experienced Non-Executive Director with a demonstrated history of working in the consumer goods industry.

321 This industry professional wishes to keep personal and company information anonymous.

Franck Moison capitalized on the importance of heritage within a brand and even the ingredients in the brand. For example, at Colgate-Palmolive he noticed the following regional and cultural nuances. Franck mentioned that Russians, generally speaking, love having medicinal herbs from the mountains in their toothpaste. In addition, he said that in India, a large number of people from India really enjoyed a toothpaste made with a plant that has been around for centuries in Ayurvedic Medicine. The toothpaste tasted familiar to them and the color of it was brown. It was a huge success in India, but this toothpaste in other regions of the world would have never worked.

Franck Moison lays it out clearly. It is imperative to adapt the global offering to a local culture. To win in the industry today, you need to be close to the consumer and marry your brand's mission to each region's heritage. Nothing ismore special than feeling like the essence of a product is made for you and your people.

Like Frank Moison, Olivier Lechére[322] shares that the medium in which you communicate your story is just as important. You must nail social media communication. New

---

322 Olivier Lechère is the General Director for Chanel Spain & Portugal in charge of the three divisions: Fashion, Fragrance & Beauty and Watches & Fine Jewelry in Madrid. He has dedicated these last twenty years to driving and growing the business by setting up two fashion flagship stores, boosting the fragrances and beauty division to number one in the Spanish market.

beauty brands form 25 percent of the market, according to Olivier Lechére, and are starting to seduce new consumers due to their positioning, new messages oriented toward environment, corporate social responsibility, naturality etc...

Olivier Lechére considers that the well-established brands are moving to a new way of communicating with their customers. He mentioned that in his case, Chanel is pushing for better consumer engagement on social media platforms. "This is our challenge for the near future," Olivier says. Chanel has dominated storytelling since the beginning of the brand's life about a century ago and now must work to maintain their storytelling to the consumers of this new era. "We have so much to tell, that if we don't tell it effectively, we become like the rest," Oliver remarks.

We need to transform the purchasing behavior in a real customer experience, nourished by the values of the brand and our own DNA. The customer needs to perceive that you are different.

The top beauty conglomerates remain relevant internationally because they very clearly follow these two formats in adaptation when telling their stories. The Vice President of Global Marketing[323] at a world leading beauty company explains how the Global Marketing team and Local Marketing work

---

323 This industry professional wishes to keep personal and company information anonymous.

and complement each other to execute peak performance for brands in their large beauty conglomerate.

1. **Global Marketing team:** They keep a uniformity in the DNA, mission, and values of a brand. It is already hard to keep the DNA of a brand with segments of it in all parts of the world. Without them making sure all the regions had the correct vision, the brand would not be successful.

2. **Local Marketing team:** The local marketing then adapts the DNA and central story/stories of the brand to a local region and culture. They take after the direction of the Global marketing team and make sure it is in a consumable and representative form in Egypt, China, etc... for the consumers to receive a message that will resonate with them.

Care for a Cause Your Consumer Cares About

Shadoh Punnapuzha[324] noted that staying close to your consumer and being present in causes they care about, but also being authentic about it, will help you in client retention. It's taking responsibility, not because it's trendy, but because it's

---

324 Shadoh Punnapuzha is the Founder of Taïla Skincare. She is proving that when you combine the power of Ayurveda and science, you get divine results. After years of working at a PE firm in NYC and going through a burnout, Shadoh found her path to a healthy life and a healthy skin through Ayurveda.

the right thing to do. You actually build your loyalty base, not only with the quality, efficacy, or effectiveness of your products, but also, with forming a tie with the social causes your brand cares about.

Influencer Marketing

People are beginning to trust mega-influencers less and less. The industry is catching on to the power of micro-influencers, who usually are more genuine with their followers. They are rarely paid for what they promote, and their followers have a strong attachment to them because they feel identified. However, for big messages to be passed on, the mega-influencers are still the ones to go to. They really have the power and the following to make a whole influx of society lean toward a certain cause or trend—think Kylie Jenner and her effect on the lip enhancement trend.[325]

There are many ways you can approach influencer marketing; you just need to make sure your approach aligns with your brand.

---

325 Witt, Natalie. 2018. "The Influence Kylie Jenner Has In Forwarding Ideologies About Body Image." *The Body Bible*. Accessed October 2 2019. http://www.blogs2018.buprojects.uk/nataliewitt/the-kylie-jenner-influence/.

Alessia Vettesse, a Harvard Business MBA student (2017-2019), studied the effectiveness of influencer marketing through celebrity endorsements and company ads for beauty consumers. The beauty consumers surveyed said they did not fully *feel* represented until influencer marketing. They did not find that previous marketing was made for them nor their skin type. Alessia Vettese concludes, "Beauty companies should create products and enlist influencers that reach people with a variety of ethnicities, skin tones, and skin sensitivities."[326]

The lessons from Vettese's research don't apply solely to beauty brands, but to other industries as well. She says, "Figure out which social media channels will attract your audience, be deliberate about how you showcase your products on different channels, and make sure the people who represent your company will be seen as authentic, trusted voices of the image you want to present."[327]

Consumers are strongly drawn to influencers who speak to them as if they were their best friends, go through life in a way they do, or have the same struggles they do or did. Since we spend a large part of our days following what these

---

326 "Lipstick Tips: How Influencers Are Making Over Beauty Marketing." 2019. HBS Working Knowledge. Accessed October 2 2019. https://hbswk.hbs.edu/item/lipstick-tips-how-influencers-are-making-over-beauty-marketing?cid=spmailing-28788595-WK percent20Newsletter percent2008-28-2019 percent20(1)-August percent2028, percent202019.

327 Ibid.

influencers tell us on social media, what they post, the places they frequent, and the products they use, we immediately turn to them for experiences.

Agility in Digital

"Although the great majority of prestige beauty sales still take place in department stores, pharmacies, and specialty stores, digital channels have become the primary arena for consumer decision-making,"[328] according to a study on the beauty industry done by Deloitte.

Jordana Shiau:[329]

> I think indie brands are rising and outperforming established brands because indie brands have more agility in the market. They're able to launch things faster and that's more relevant to the beauty consumer. Indie brands don't have layers of approvals or forecasting they can just launch. I think the industry

---

328 2019. *Www2.Deloitte.Com*. Accessed October 2 2019. https://www2.deloitte.com/content/dam/Deloitte/cn/Documents/international-business-support/deloitte-cn-ibs-france-beauty-market-en-2017.pdf.

329 Jordana Shiau is a Manager of Social and Digital Strategy at Laura Mercier. She has been in the corporate side of the beauty industry for the last five years working from startups to the largest beauty brands in the world.

is changing so much and the demand for things is growing so much that you have to be agile to make it.

ColourPop Cosmetics is a good example because they have been successful in launching products like nobody's business. They do not have anyone holding them back. They can see something trending and immediately launch it at an affordable price.

Point of Sale User Experience (UX)

Although the focus on digital is important, we need to maximize all channels where the consumer can be found. Older demographics watch more TV and less Instagram. Therefore for some products, a more traditional form of marketing can work as well.

Other experiential mediums to look at in beauty are airports, air travel, and other travel retail space. Today's generation turns to travel and experience as the "go-to leisure," and thus it becomes the most valuable point of sale location. A big conglomerate executive points to beautiful stores in airports as great communication tools for brands. This is especially the case for beauty products as there is a greater chance for consumers to purchase in person as they can experience the product and test it out themselves before purchasing—allowing the product to appeal to the senses, not only seen through the medium of a silver screen.

IS TOO SATURATED A BAD THING?

Ultimately, having more beauty brands in the market is creating more opportunities for consumers to buy products suited for them and makes them *feel* more beautiful.

"Currently, there is a lot out there, but the point of all the brands is to complement each other and focus on all the consumer needs. Social media is making it easier for there to be more awareness and communication between both sides," says the Marketing Director of the Americas beauty division at a luxury goods company.[330]

However, in the long-run, the same the Marketing Director states, "I think smaller brands are taking up a lot of market share. They are a lot more agile, but they will not be as relevant as the more established conglomerates in the long-run, especially as the large beauty houses are creating a diversified portfolio that is covering a more and more wholesome definition of beauty."

No matter if you are a small or large brand, focus on these two things:

1. Stay true to your brand DNA and values even when you innovate.

---

330 This industry professional wishes to keep personal and company information anonymous.

2. All companies need to be on their toes. The best way to do that is with direct consumer engagement.

Consumers are savvy and know where to source what and from which brand. If they want to buy a skin care or makeup staple, they will go to a large key brand, but if they want something "fun," they will probably go to a more dynamic and versatile indie name. I believe both the foundational beauty brands and newer more niche brands complement each other and balance each other out.

If you look at what is happening in the market, consumers want to try new brands with a totally different personality. Beauty conglomerates, such as L'Oréal, Estée Lauder, Shiseido, and Coty have caught on and are acquiring many indie brands to complete their circle of beauty. Entrepreneurs have been launching more niche brands to fill in the untapped potential of the market. All with one purpose—to allow consumers to *feel* cared for, loved, and put forth the most beautiful versions of ourselves. This is a very exciting moment in the beauty industry.

Due to the nature of competition and the talk around beauty, achieving success in the industry has become increasingly unpredictable, especially with the number of new entrants in the market. According to a study by Deloitte "As many as 90 percent of beauty product launches fail within a year."[331]

Professionals, work hard, keep your clients' beauty as your number one priority, and succeed!

WHAT CONSTITUTES SUCCESS?

Olga Lorencin[332] identifies six ways a beauty company, brand, or line can claim success:

- Consistent high ratings across your platforms
- Consumer loyalty
- Being acquired—having something so special that a more powerful and influential brand wants to buy you
- Products that continuously perform well
- Products showing results—questionable how to measures "results," but some brands are clear about how they show them
- Longevity of a product(s) if you have been around for a long time

---

331 2019. *Www2.Deloitte.Com.* Accessed October 2 2019. https://
www2.deloitte.com/content/dam/Deloitte/cn/Documents/
international-business-support/deloitte-cn-ibs-france-beauty-
market-en-2017.pdf.

332 Olga Lorencin is the owner of Olga Lorencin Skin Care Clinic
and CEO and founder for Olga Lorencin Skin Care. She is a
top-tier esthetician and skin care guru and has spent more than
twenty years in the treatment room studying ingredients. Olga is
affectionately referred to as "The Acid Queen."

Important to Keep in Mind, A Checklist:

Key Points from Dr. John Martin on the Cosmetic Industry and Skin Care:[333]

- Try to find something new or different that can help with skin rejuvenation but make sure it actually works.
- New formulations of time-proven ingredients such as Retinol can be popular.
- Keep regimens simple. No one wants to do a ten-step process.
- Most people have realized that outrageous prices for products do not mean they are any better. Keep it reasonable.

Key Take-Aways Checklist:

- Stay true to the DNA of your brand.
- Keep that MAGIC alive.
- Target a niche market and stick to what your company does best.
- Disrupt the market with a cutting edge or innovative idea/formula/device/treatment/product that differentiates you from the saturated market.
- Leverage results-oriented/scientifically backed products and technology.
- Be consumer-centric.

---

333 Dr. John Martin is a Harvard-educated Medical Doctor who specializes in Facial Cosmetic Surgery as well as other non-surgical treatment for vascular and pigment problems as well as skinrejuvenation. Dr. Martin has been featured in *The Doctors, The Dr. Oz Show, Dr. Phil,* and *Anderson Cooper 360°.*

- Use social media and experiences as medium(s) to tell your story. Keep it consistent.
- Relate to your consumers' identity, gender, ethnicity, background, but more importantly their lifestyle.
- Engage with your consumers and listen to their needs.
- Care for what consumers care for. Educate, inspire and promote social good.
- Stay on top of trends.
- Commit to your brand.
- Do your homework.
- Work hard toward your brand and your mission.
- Work because you love it.
- Work because it's your life.

EPILOGUE

—

"What is beauty? An idea, a feeling, a pleasure, an emotion. And yet a mystery at the same time. Beauty, like time, is something no one truly understands. No definition can ever fully capture beauty."

—JEAN D'ORMESSON, *GUIDE DES ÉGARES*[334]

We are at an exciting point in the history of the beauty industry. It is becoming a safe space for everyone to celebrate their unique beauty, practice self-care, and really engage in "me-time." We are being provided more tools than ever before to internalize who we are and what mark we want to leave behind.

—

334 Ormesson, Jean d'. *Guide des égarés* Paris: Gallimard, 2016.

At the same time, the threat of information overload is on the rise. We have so much at our fingertips due to influencers and the hype surrounding health, beauty, and wellness. Now, we can access information and influence what the next individual perceives. They, in turn, pass it onto others in the expanding social network. We have all become advocates for what we think but not all advocates are well informed.

Today's beauty industry is becoming a bridge for all those who have felt marginalized from the conversation. Beauty is now being translated more as a form of self-expression, and one that is fluid between gender and ethnicities. It is our duty as citizens of the world to seek beauty in ourselves and see a world beyond our own. If you want to be celebrated by others, you must first celebrate yourself and all that constitutes you.

Whether it's a serum, face mask, moisturizer, oil massage, blush, red lipstick, or anything really that makes an individual *feel* like they are going to seize the day, the beauty industry can empower current and future generations to be a better version of themselves. I encourage you to be a more alert and conscious consumer.

Time passes, and trends fluctuate, but people's desire to engage with the beauty industry never wavers. Underneath it all is the human need not only to look beautiful but also to *feel* beautiful especially in times such as these, when lives are busy and often in solitude.

Find your beauty, your voice, and your authentic twist. That is why people will remember you. That spark you have, whether it be intellectual, emotional, behavioral, or even something you may consider a defect or imperfection can be endearing to a stranger. That is where beauty lies.

Let's not forget that we are all human. It's okay to not *feel* your best from time to time, to be stressed and to be overwhelmed. In these times life tests you. They say, when it rains, it pours, and when it does, it is almost impossible to see our beauty from within because we are looking outward through a blurred lens. However, in these instances you must make the extra effort to *feel* beautiful, for your own sake.

In the last few months of composing this book, I was in the most beautiful city in the world, Paris, and yet my eyes were glued to the computer screen, making sure I delivered my best work. Some family matters got in the way and unexpected sources of stress came about. Yet again, this is normal. Here existed a great opportunity to practice what I preach in my own book.

Have a holistic approach to your beauty. It is not about the quick fixes. It is about how you care for yourself now, tomorrow, and the day after. This is beauty, an expression of your identity, your self-love, your health and wellness, your wisdom, and your love for others. Cherish yourself, your friends, your neighbors, strangers, and put a smile on that face through the good and soon-to-be-better times.

You are radiating already.

Feel it.

You are beautiful.

WORKS REFERENCED

———

Chapter 1 — We All Want to Be Beautiful

"Cleopatra's Eye: The Significance of Kohl in Ancient Egypt." 2018. The Recipes Project. Accessed September 30, 2019. https://recipes.hypotheses.org/12837.

Fitoussi, Michèle, Bignold, Kate, and Ramakrishnan Iyer, Lakshmi. *Helena Rubinstein: The Woman Who Invented Beauty*. London, Great Britain: Gallic Books, 2013.

"History of Makeup | History of Cosmetics | BH Cosmetics LLC." 2019. BH Cosmetics. Accessed September 30, 2019. https://www.bhcosmetics.com/pages/resources-makeup-and-cosmetics-history.

Sava, Sanda. 2016. "A History of Make-Up & Fashion: 1900-1910 - Sanda Sava | Make-Up Artist." Sanda Sava | Make-Up Artist. Accessed September 30, 2019. https://sandasava.com/beauty-style/a-history-of-make-up-fashion-1900-1910/.

"The History of Beauty." 2010. HBS Working Knowledge. Accessed September 30, 2019. https://hbswk.hbs.edu/item/the-history-of-beauty.

Chapter 2 — YOUR Perception of Beauty

Martin, Gary. 2019. "'Beauty Is In The Eye Of The Beholder'—The Meaning And Origin Of This Phrase." https://www.phrases.org.uk/meanings/beauty-is-in-the-eye-of-the-beholder.html.

Ormesson, Jean d'. *Guide des égarés* Paris: Gallimard, 2016.

Chapter 3 — Subconsciously Subscribing to Trends, Behaviors, and Expectations

2019. *Dove.Com*. Accessed October 4 2019. https://www.dove.com/us/en/stories/about-dove/our-research.html.

"Lady Gaga And The Power Of Makeup For Allure Magazine | Tom + Lorenzo." 2019. Tom + Lorenzo. Accessed September 30, 2019. https://tomandlorenzo.com/2019/09/lady-gaga-for-allure-magazine-beauty-issue/.

"New Guidelines Redefine Birth Years for Millennials, Gen-X, And 'Post-Millennials'." 2018. *Mentalfloss.Com*. Accessed October 4 2019. http://mentalfloss.com/article/533632/new-guidelines-redefine-birth-years-millennials-gen-x-and-post-millennials.

Chapter 4 — Including All in The Conversation

Agren, David. 2018. "'We Can Do It': Yalitza Aparicio'S Vogue Cover Hailed By Indigenous Women." *The Guardian*. Accessed October 1 2019. https://www.theguardian.com/film/2018/dec/21/yalitza-aparicio-vogue-mexico-cover-roma-indigenous.

Beauty Is More Diverse Than Ever. But Is It Diverse Enough?." 2019. Nytimes.Com. Accessed October 1 2019. https://www.nytimes.com/2018/09/11/style/beauty-diversity.html.

"From 4000 BCE To Today: The Fascinating History of Men And Makeup." 2019. *Byrdie*. Accessed October 1 2019. https://www.byrdie.com/history-makeup-gender#targetText=For percent20millenniapercent2C percent

"Here's the Important Reason Sephora Is Closing All Its Stores For An Hour On June 5." 2019. *Bustle*. Accessed October 1 2019. https://www.bustle.com/p/sephoras-we-belong-to-something-beautiful-pledge-further-proves-the-brands-commitment-to-diversity-17911715.

"Isabella Rossellini Returns to Lancôme." 2016. *Fashionnetwork.Com*. Accessed October 1 2019. https://ww.fashionnetwork.com/news/Isabella-Rossellini-returns-to-Lancome,665917.html#.XXPTui2B124.

"North America: Mexico—The World Factbook—Central Intelligence Agency." 2019. *Cia.Gov*. Accessed October 1 2019. https://www.cia.gov/library/publications/the-world-factbook/geos/print_mx.html.

Number of Smartphone Users Worldwide 2014-2020 | Statista." 2019. *Statista*. Accessed October 1 2019. https://www.statista.com/statistics/330695/number-of-smartphone-users-worldwide/.

"Rising Gender-Neutral Brands—Cosmetic Executive Women." 2019. Cosmetic Executive Women. Accessed October 8 2019. https://www.cew.org/beauty_news/rising-gender-neutral-brands/.

Size, Full, Full Size, Full Size, and BUSINESS WIRE. 2019. "Pantene Launches 'Don't Hate Me Because I'M #Beautifulgbtq' To Redefine What 'Beautiful' Looks Like Today." *Businesswire.Com*. Accessed October 1 2019. https://www.businesswire.com/news/home/20190618005209/en/.

Stuart, Eden. 2019. "Sephora Commits To Inclusivity With Platform, Manifesto." *Global Cosmetic Industry*. Accessed October 1 2019. https://www.gcimagazine.com/marketstrends/channels/other/Sephora-Commits-to-Inclusivity-with-Platform-Manifesto-510510391.html.

"The History of Beauty." 2010. *HBS Working Knowledge*. Accessed September 30, 2019. https://hbswk.hbs.edu/item/the-history-of-beauty.

"The History of Male Makeup." 2012. *Infashuationdotnet.Wordpress.Com*. Accessed October 1 2019. https://infashuationdotnet.wordpress.com/2012/12/07/mens-makeup/.

"Tribe Dynamics: Top Indie Brands Of Q2 2019—Cosmetic Executive Women." 2019. Cosmetic Executive Women. *Accessed November 3 2019. https://www.cew.org/beauty_news/tribe-dynamics-indie-beauty-debrief-for-q2-2019/*.

Warfield, Nia. 2019. "Men Are A Multibillion Dollar Growth Opportunity For The Beauty Industry." *CNBC*. Accessed October 1 2019. https://www.cnbc.com/2019/05/17/men-are-a-multibillion-dollar-growth-opportunity-for-the-beauty-industry.html.

"Yalitza Aparicio En La Portada De Vogue México—Enero 2019." 2019. *YouTube*. Accessed October 1 2019. https://www.youtube.com/watch?v=SmEhcDZqrUo.

"Yalitza Aparicio Is On The 2019 TIME 100 List | Time.Com." 2019. Time.Com. *Accessed August 1 2019. https://time.com/collection/100-most-influential-people-2019/5567863/yalitza-aparicio/*.

Chapter 5 — Connecting with Yourself and The Right Ingredients

"7 Apps To Help You Check For Chemicals & Find Non-Toxic Alternatives." 2019. Tox Free Family. Accessed October 6 2019. https://toxfreefamily.com/mobile-apps-to-reduce-harsh-chemical-exposure/.

"Benefits of Yoga | American Osteopathic Association." 2019. *American Osteopathic Association*. Accessed October 6 2019. https://osteopathic.org/ what-is-osteopathic-medicine/benefits-of-yoga/.

Brazier, Yvette, and MS Yamini Ranchod. 2017. "Acupuncture: How It Works, Uses, Benefits, And Risks." Medical News Today. *Accessed October 6 2019. https://www.medicalnewstoday.com/articles/156488.php.*

"FDA Authority Over Cosmetics: How Cosmetics Are Not FDA-Approved." 2019. *U.S. Food And Drug Administration*. Accessed October 6 2019. https:// www.fda.gov/cosmetics/cosmetics-laws-regulations/fda-authority-over-cosmetics-how-cosmetics-are-not-fda-approved-are-fda-regulated.

"I Tried Oil Pulling For (Almost) A Week: Here's What Happened." 2019. Fashionista. *Accessed October 6 2019.* https://fashionista.com/2014/03/oil-pulling.

Lallanilla, Marc. 2015. "Ayurveda: Facts About Ayurvedic Medicine." Livescience. Com. *Accessed October 6 2019. https://www.livescience.com/42153-ayurveda.html#targetText=Ayurveda percent20is percent20an percent20ancientpercent20health,)percent20andpercent20veda percent20(knowledge.*

Newman, Tim, and OD Ann Marie Griff. 2017. "Reiki: What Is It And Are There Benefits?" Medical News Today. *Accessed October 6 2019.* https://www.medicalnewstoday.com/articles/308772.php.

"Pranayama | Ekhart Yoga." 2019. *Ekhartyoga.Com*. Accessed October 6 2019. https://www.ekhartyoga.com/resources/styles/pranayama.

The Beauty Closet | Goop. 2019. Goop. Accessed October 6 2019. https://goop. com/beauty-closet-podcast/.

"The Goop Podcast: Feeding Your Digestive Fire On Apple Podcasts." *2019. Apple Podcasts. Accessed November 4 2019.* https://podcasts.apple.com/bs/ podcast/feeding-your-digestive-fire/id1352546554?i=1000447315789.

"THE GREEN BAROMETER SURVEY." 2019. *Kari Gran Skin Care*. Accessed October 6 2019. https://karigran.com/pages/the-green-barometer-survey.

"The Personal Care Product Safety Act." 2019. EWG. Accessed November 4 2019. https://www.ewg.org/personalcareproductsafetyact.

"These 5 Apps Tell You What's In Your Beauty Products So You Can Shop Safer." 2019. Bustle. *Accessed October 6 2019. https://www.bustle.com/p/5-apps-that-tell-you-whats-in-beauty-products-because-knowledge-is-power-11997650.*

"Tribe Dynamics: August'S Top 10 Cosmetics, Skin Care And Hair Brands On Social—Cosmetic Executive Women." 2019. Cosmetic Executive Women. *Accessed November 3 2019. https://www.cew.org/beauty_news/ tribe-dynamics-augusts-top-10-cosmetics-skin-care-and-hair-brands-on-social/.*

"What Is Ayurveda?—National Ayurvedic Medical Association." 2019. National Ayurvedic Medical Association. Accessed October 6 2019. https://www. ayurvedanama.org/what-is-ayurveda.

"What Is Greenwashing?—Definition From Whatis.Com." 2019. Whatis.Com. Accessed October 6 2019. https://whatis.techtarget.com/definition/greenwashing.

"Why Are There Still Toxic Ingredients In Beauty Products? | Goop." 2019. Goop. Accessed October 6 2019. https://goop.com/beauty-closet-podcast/ why-are-there-still-toxic-ingredients-in-beauty-products/.

WIRE, BUSINESS. 2019. "Global $4.6 Billion Collagen Market by Product Type, Source, Application and Region—Forecast To 2023—Researchandmarkets.Com." *Businesswire.Com.* Accessed October 6 2019. https://www.businesswire.com/news/ home/20190308005227/en/Global-4.6-Billion-Collagen-Market-Product-Type.

Zanolli, Lauren. 2019. "Pretty Hurts: Are Chemicals In Beauty Products Making Us Ill?" *The Guardian.* Accessed October 6 2019. https://www.theguardian.com/ us-news/2019/may/23/are-chemicals-in-beauty-products-making-us-ill.

Chapter 6 — Influenced to be a "Hackable Human"

2019. *Linqia.Com.* Accessed October 2 2019. https://linqia.com/wp-content/ uploads/2019/04/Linqia-State-of-Influencer-Marketing-2019-Report.pdf.

"Dr. Few: A Plastic Surgeon On Going Little (Not Big) | Goop." 2019. *Goop.* Accessed November 6 2019. https://goop.com/beauty-closet-podcast/ dr-few-a-plastic-surgeon-on-going-little-not-big/.

Harari, Yuval. 2018. "Why Technology Favors Tyranny." The Atlantic. Accessed November 3 2019. https://www.theatlantic.com/magazine/archive/2018/10/ yuval-noah-harari-technology-tyranny/568330/.

Harari, Yuval N. *21 Lessons for the 21st Century* London: Jonathan Cape, 2018.

"INFLUENCER MARKETING 2019: Why Brands Can't Get Enough Of An $8 Billion Ecosystem Driven By Kardashians, Moms, And Tweens." 2019. Business Insider France. *Accessed November 5 2019. https://www.businessinsider.fr/us/ the-2019-influencer-marketing-report-2019-7.*

Mueffling, C. (n.d.). *Ageless Beauty the French Way*. 1st ed. New York City: St. Martin's Press, 2018. p.14.

Nast, Condé. 2018. "Everything You've Ever Wanted To Know About Fillers." *Allure*. Accessed October 3 2019. https://www.allure.com/story/facial-fillers-information-guide.

Nast, Condé. 2019. "The 7 Plastic Surgery Trends That Will Be Huge This Year." *Allure*. Accessed November 6 2019. https://www.allure.com/story/plastic-surgery-procedure-trends-2019.

Pearl, Diana, and Diana Pearl. 2019. "75 percent Of Estée Lauder's Marketing Budget Is Going To Digital—And Influencers." *Adweek.Com*. Accessed October 2 2019. https://www.adweek.com/brand-marketing/75-of-estee-lauders-marketing-budget-is-going-to-influencers/.

"The Angelababy Effect: More Women Want Double Eyelid Like Actress." 2017. *South China Morning Post*. Accessed October 3 2019. https://www.scmp.com/lifestyle/health-beauty/article/2093921/why-double-eyelid-surgery-rise-asia-rising-incomes-and.

"This Is How Much Instagram Influencers Really Cost." 2019. *Later Blog*. Accessed October 2 2019. https://later.com/blog/instagram-influencers-costs/.

The Top Beauty and Makeup Artist Influencers Of 2019." 2019. *IZEA*. Accessed October 2 2019. https://izea.com/2019/02/01/makeup-artist/.

"Why More Women Are Happily Going Without Makeup." 2019. Psychology Today. *Accessed October 2 2019. https://www.psychologytoday.com/ca/blog/the-clarity/201707/why-more-women-are-happily-going-without-makeup.*

Chapter 7 — Honor Yourself

Chinwe Esimai, "The African Woman Leading Citi's Anti-Bribery & Corruption Efforts." 2019. *Facebook Watch*. Accessed October 3 2019. https://www.facebook.com/Face2FaceAfrica/videos/836609520007529/?v=836609520007529.

"Why More Women Are Happily Going Without Makeup." 2019. Psychology Today. Accessed October 2 2019. https://www.psychologytoday.com/ca/blog/the-clarity/201707/why-more-women-are-happily-going-without-makeup.

Chapter 8 — Power of Unique Beauty

"A Quote by Coco Chanel." 2019. Goodreads.Com. Accessed October 6 2019. https://www.goodreads.com/ quotes/7121021-beauty-begins-the-moment-you-decide-to-be-yourself.

"Dr. Few: A Plastic Surgeon On Going Little (Not Big) | Goop." 2019. *Goop*. Accessed November 6 2019. https://goop.com/beauty-closet-podcast/ dr-few-a-plastic-surgeon-on-going-little-not-big/.

Mueffling, C. (n.d.). *Ageless Beauty the French Way*. 1st ed. New York City: St. Martin's Press, 2018. p.14.

Nast, Condé. 2018. "Everything You've Ever Wanted To Know About Fillers." *Allure*. Accessed October 3 2019. https://www.allure.com/story/ facial-fillers-information-guide.

Nast, Condé. 2019. "The 7 Plastic Surgery Trends That Will Be Huge This Year." *Allure*. Accessed November 6 2019. https://www.allure.com/story/ plastic-surgery-procedure-trends-2019.

"The Angelababy Effect: More Women Want Double Eyelid Like Actress." 2017. *South China Morning Post*. Accessed October 3 2019. https://www.scmp.com/lifestyle/health-beauty/article/2093921/ why-double-eyelid-surgery-rise-asia-rising-incomes-and.

"Why More Women Are Happily Going Without Makeup." 2019. *Psychology Today*. Accessed October 3 2019. https://www.psychologytoday.com/ca/blog/ the-clarity/201707/why-more-women-are-happily-going-without-makeup.

Chapter 9 — Three Beauties Making a Difference in a Sector They Didn't Expect

"Doctor And Team." 2019. *Dr-Barbara-Sturm.Com*. Accessed September 1 2019. https://www.dr-barbara-sturm.com/clinic/doctor-and-team/.

"Dr. Barbara Sturm Has Bottled The Fountain Of Youth." 2019. *Forbes.Com*. Accessed October 10 2019. https:// www.forbes.com/sites/addiewagenknecht/2018/05/08/ dr-barbara-sturm-is-changing-how-we-age-or-dont/#68a726ef5eca.

Nast, Condé. 2016. "This Scientist And Beauty Guru's 9-To-5 Style Isn't Limited to A Lab Coat." Vogue. Accessed October 10 2019. *https://www.vogue.com/article/ barbara-sturm-cher-angela-bassett-kim-kardashian-west-beauty-scientist*.

Chapter 10 — Becoming a Smarter Beauty Consumer

"Why Are There Still Toxic Ingredients In Beauty Products? | Goop." 2019. *Goop.* Accessed October 6 2019. https://goop.com/beauty-closet-podcast/why-are-there-still-toxic-ingredients-in-beauty-products/.

Chapter 11 — Success in Your Beauty Business

2019. *Www2.Deloitte.Com.* Accessed October 2 2019. https://www2.deloitte.com/content/dam/Deloitte/cn/Documents/international-business-support/deloitte-cn-ibs-france-beauty-market-en-2017.pdf.

"Huffpost Is Now A Part Of Verizon Media." 2019. Huffpost. Com. *Accessed November 7 2019. https://www.huffpost.com/entry/estee-lauder-quotes-beauty-business_n_3506334.*

"Lipstick Tips: How Influencers Are Making Over Beauty Marketing." 2019. HBS Working Knowledge. Accessed October 2 2019. https://hbswk.hbs.edu/item/lipstick-tips-how-influencers-are-making-over-beauty-marketing?cid=spmailing-28788595-WK percent20Newsletter percent2008-28-2019 percent20(1)-August percent2028, percent202019.

Witt, Natalie. 2018. "The Influence Kylie Jenner Has In Forwarding Ideologies About Body Image." *The Body Bible.* Accessed October 2 2019. http://www.blogs2018.buprojects.uk/nataliewitt/the-kylie-jenner-influence/.

ACKNOWLEDGMENTS

———

First and foremost, I would like to thank all the people I had the wonderful opportunity to meet, spend time with, and interview during my research for this book. Thank you for taking time away from your busy schedules to share all these invaluable accounts. You have made the content in this book like no other, compiling firsthand insights and stories that make us rethink what we thought was true about the beauty industry.

I want to extend my dearest gratitude to two very special women who were crucial in the formation of this book, Monica Vidal and Jackie Camacho. Because of them, I was able to speak to some of the most important professionals in the industry. Not only that, but they have played an enormous role throughout this process, giving me wholehearted support and guidance even when composing a book was simply an idea. I admire both of you and hope to open doors in the future for other hard working, giving, and inspiring individuals.

Papa, Mama, and Jimena, thank you for your unconditional love. As cliché as this will sound, you are the most important people in my life. Everything I am is because of you. Thank you for being my rock, lifting me up every time I fall, and pushing me to keep pursuing, dancing, running, living, and thriving. *No hay palabras suficientes para agradeceros todo lo que siempre habéis hecho por mi y todo lo que me habéis enseñado. Gracias por dejarme soñar y animarme a hacer realidad mis sueños.*

A huge thank you to my extraordinary friends, who accepted to be my advanced readers. I am blessed to have gotten your authentic and constructive feedback on my chapters. I am forever touched by your willingness to help, Max Lawton, Anna von Griesheim, Haley Schusterman, Sophia Waitt, Heather Van Rieper, Anne Marie Collins, Emily Devery, Olivia Salberg, Sophie Ball, Fleur Oostwal, Alanna Samarin, Nicolas Williamson, Natalie De Cesare, Rachel Brothers, Morgan Luellwitz, Emma Cappiello, Lillian Roos, and Kendal Gee. A special thanks to Lyle Li for being my right hand throughout this process.

An enormous thank you to New Degree Press' incredible team—especially Brian Bies, Heather Gomez, Leila Summers, and Eric Koester. Thank you for seeing the potential in me and being by my side every step of the way!

Last, but definitely not least, thank you to all my supporters. You have been my biggest cheerleaders all along. You gave me the motivation to keep writing in times of absolute writer's block. I am forever grateful for that.

This goes to you all; my success is your success.

MY LOVELY SUPPORTERS:

Abbey Pickett	Andrew Finnegan
Adriana Alonso	Angela Jung
Alanna Samarin	Anisha Pathak
Alejandro Freijo Benito	Anna von Griesheim
Alejandro Wiley	Anne Marie Collins
Alexandra Acosta	Anniela Achar
Alfonso Baigorri	Ariana Rodriguez-Fiol
Alicia Carabarin	Ashley Devery
Amanda Anchipolovsky	Belen Benito Gracia
Ana Allende	Camila Guyot
Andrea Prudencio	Camille Farge
Andrea Rallo	Candido Rodriguez
Andrea Stenslie	Carla Mauri

Carlos Rodriguez Aspirichaga

Carlota Sanchez

Casa Ana Gomez

Cathy Calhoun

Cheryl Hicks

Chloe Farrick

Christine Rutkowski

Conchita Calderon

Connor Niemann

Cornelia von Rittberg

Daniel Wick

Daniela Bao

Delia Rodriguez

Dinah Pourbaba

Eduardo Pelaez

Elena Del Barrio

Elena Jakubowicz

Elizabeth Benham

Emma Cappiello

Emma Howie

Eric Koester

Esteban Estevez Zurita

Ewelina Aiossa

Farah Matquez

Fleur Oostwal

Francesca Macrae

Francois Stassen

Grace Blue

Graciela Feijo Benito

Haley Schusterman

Heather Van Riper

Hector Sulaiman Saldivar

Henry Quilici

Hoda Tahoun

Hunter Pitts

Ignacio Olarra

Ioanna-India McTaggart

Iokin Azcarraga

Isabella Gradney

Jacinta Legorreta

James Lonergan

Jennifer Kopelman

Jenny Drew Garabedian

Jeronimo Garcia Moreno

Jessie Penn

Jimena Rodriguez-Benito

Jose Ignacio Jimenez Cortes

Juan Pablo Villarreal

Juana Montero

Karla Alvarez Buzali

Kelley Hawke

Kelly Fertel

Kendal Gee

Kosara Tsoneva

Lara Fares
Laura Benito Gracia
Lauren Brackmann
Lauren Hicks
Lillian Roos
Line Szegedi Jess
Loles Vica
Lorena Mercado Garde
Lorena Plaza
Luis de Antonio
Lyle Li
Mackenzie Luderer
Manu Vecino
Manuel Sanchez
Mar Hernandez
Margarita Barrero
María Calderon
Maria Florencia Culaciati
Maria Mantero
Mary Jo Luellwitz
Max Ascolani
Maxwell Waitt
McKayla Harris
Megan Plancher
Melissa Medina
Mia Marotta
Miguel Barbosa

Monica Lisazo
Monica Vidal
Morgan Luellwitz
Nadia Rodriguez
Natalia Esteve
Natalia Vazquez
Natalie De Cesare
Nicholas Goldlust
Nicholas Schlegel
Nick Metzler
Nicolas Williamson
Nina Rodriguez
Olivia Ballve
Olivia Salberg
Paola von Bertrab
Petra Wissenburg
Pierina Merino
Priyanka Agrawal
Rachel Brothers
Ramiro Gonzalez Luna
Rebecca Vangelos
Ricardo Mendez Gutierrez
Rodrigo de los Santos
Santiago Rodriguez
Sebastian Williamson
Silvia Bermudez
Silvia Navascues

Skye Lucas
Skyler Baldwin
Sofia Olarra
Sophia Ball
Sophia Stallone
Sophia Waitt
Stella Lo Balbo
Susana de Eusebio

Taylor Leah Singer
Taylor Sui
Teresa Gaya
Tomas Diez Canedo Carrasco
Valentina Maio
Viviana Du Pond
Wanda Lima
Yolanda Benito Gracia

Made in the USA
Columbia, SC
29 December 2019